"Every woman concerned about her health or the health of the women in her life should read *Your Healthiest Healthy*. It's like talking to an extremely knowledgeable girlfriend. Samantha has done her homework and offers so much great understanding, perspective, and realistic advice. She isn't afraid to hold back, but she still knows how to have a good time. **This book will change your life!**"

—**KRIS JENNER**, bestselling author of *Kris Jenner . . . and All Things Kardashian* and *In the Kitchen with Kris*

"What a great read! *Your Healthiest Healthy* is equally entertaining and enlightening and for newbies and health nuts alike. I especially love how Samantha breaks everything down into small steps to make it all accessible to everyone. **This is such an incredible resource for all-around healthy living.**"

—**BROOKE BURKE**, TV host, wellness guru, author and creator of *Brooke Burke Body*, and CEO of ModernMom.com

"*Your Healthiest Healthy* is pragmatic and encyclopedic in scope, and I love that it approaches health from so many insightful angles: biological, emotional, interpersonal, and spiritual. **This well-researched book features so much great practical advice** for anyone who wants to maintain intimate relationships, manage risk for chronic diseases, and live a healthier life."

—**DREW PINSKY**, MD, internist/addictionologist, and bestselling author of *The Mirror Effect*

"**This eye-opening and empowering guide** provides the essential road map for anyone dealing with a health crisis. It's comprehensive yet conversational, and it **will help you live your best, healthiest life every day.**"

—**CHRISTINA APPLEGATE**, Emmy® Award–winning actress, founder of Right Action for Women, and cancer survivor

"I'm blown away. What a great thing to put out into the world. **If knowledge is power, then Samantha Harris is Wonder Woman.** In this book, she has gathered detailed information to give women going through breast cancer a way to take positive control of their situation, from what products or chemicals to avoid to how to find new ways to live a healthy lifestyle through positivity. Samantha shows that you can live a better life even after a shocking diagnosis. Give this book to anyone going through breast cancer and at any stage after. This is going to do so much good for so many women. **What an amazingly fabulous book!**"

—**RITA WILSON**, actress, producer, winner of the Producers Guild of America Visionary Award, and breast cancer survivor

"No matter how many times life knocks you down, it takes strength and perseverance to get back up and fight. *Your Healthiest Healthy* gives you the power to do just that with great stories and helpful tips. Whether you need a little pick me up or a total health overhaul, **this invaluable book will transform you into a bona fide fighter** and make you feel like a champion."

—**LAILA ALI**, super middleweight and light heavyweight boxing champion and author of *Reach!* and *Food for Life*

"*Your Healthiest Healthy* is **a shot of pure inspiration.** Samantha's powerful, witty journey from cancer diagnosis to hilarious missteps to full recovery **is a must-read.** It's real, relatable, and research-backed. I strongly recommend it for any woman who wants to make smarter choices for her health. *Your Healthiest Healthy* is a page-turner that **will turn your life around.**"

—**RACHEL BELLER**, RDN, bestselling author, and CEO of Beller Nutrition Institute

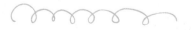

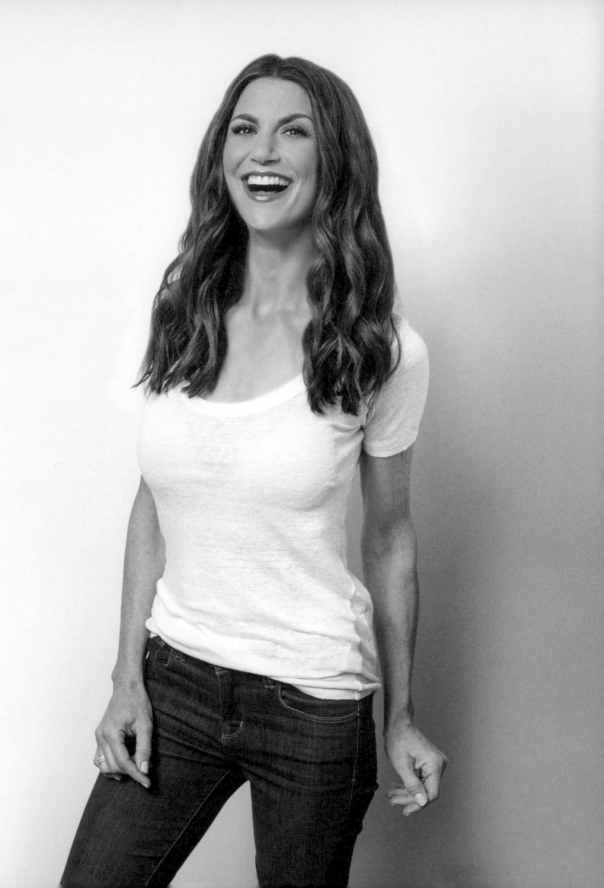

Your Healthiest Healthy

8 EASY WAYS to Take Control, Help Prevent AND Fight Cancer, AND Live a Longer, Cleaner, Happier Life

SAMANTHA HARRIS

STERLING
New York

STERLING
New York

An Imprint of Sterling Publishing Co., Inc.
1166 Avenue of the Americas
New York, NY 10036

ISBN 978-1-4549-2892-8

Distributed in Canada by Sterling Publishing Co., Inc.
C/o Canadian Manda Group, 664 Annette Street
Toronto, Ontario, M6S 2C8, Canada
Distributed in the United Kingdom by GMC Distribution Services
Castle Place, 166 High Street, Lewes, East Sussex, BN7 1XU, United Kingdom
Distributed in Australia by NewSouth Books
45 Beach Street, Coogee, NSW 2034, Australia

For information about custom editions, special sales, and premium and corporate purchases,
please contact Sterling Special Sales at 800-805-5489 or specialsales@sterlingpublishing.com.

Manufactured in China

2 4 6 8 10 9 7 5 3 1

sterlingpublishing.com
samantha-harris.com
yourhealthiesthealthy.com

Cover design by Elizabeth Mihaltse Lindy
Interior design by Christine Heun

For image credits, see page 207.

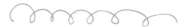

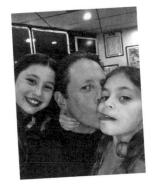

For my loves who are my life,
Michael, Jossie, and Hilly.
Because of and for you, I am
inspired to be my healthiest
self and to help you do the same.

For my mom, Bonnie, and my sister,
Aimée, because you both love all of me and
challenge me always to be my best self.

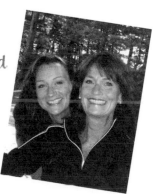

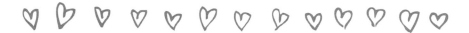

CONTENTS

FOREWORD

As a medical oncologist, I have the privilege and responsibility of interacting with people during one of the most important events in their lives: a new diagnosis of cancer. Their reactions and concerns are as diverse as they are, but some approaches remain common to everyone facing this challenge. Initial questions focus around three major areas:

1. Prognosis: Can I be cured? Will I need to learn to live with this disease as a chronic illness? Will I die from it?
2. Treatment: What's the treatment plan for my disease? How will that treatment impact my life, work, family, and friends?
3. My Role: What can I do, beyond the role of patient, to help in the treatment of my disease?

Samantha Harris addresses that third question in great depth in this book.

She and I met in 2014 when, as a host for *Entertainment Tonight*, she interviewed me about *Living Proof*, a made-for-TV movie starring Harry Connick Jr., playing me, that tells the story of the making of a new breast cancer drug. At that time, I had been doing basic research and clinically practicing medical oncology for some 25 years, and my lab helped discover HER2-positive breast cancer, an important subset of the disease, and also helped in developing Herceptin, a new targeted therapy to treat it.

During our conversation, Samantha shared that she had just faced the challenge of a new breast cancer diagnosis herself. After I discussed the work that my lab had been doing and she told me about her own case, she entrusted her care to my clinic. Her drive, sharp intellect, and intense interest in doing everything she could to improve her health and play an active role in the treatment of her disease struck me immediately. She read about breast cancer voraciously and always asked insightful questions about her case and her treatment plan. She also asked a lot about other subtypes of the disease and about cancer and cancer care in general. She was extremely inquisitive, consistently well-informed, and always dynamically engaged.

Samantha's experiences and how she handled them form the basis for *Your Healthiest Healthy*. In the pages that follow, she takes you carefully and thoughtfully through the steps that she took in meeting the challenge of her own diagnosis. She was 40 years old at the time and in otherwise "perfect" health with a great personal fitness level. She had a healthy lifestyle and no significant family history of cancer. Yet here she sat with a new diagnosis of breast cancer. How could this be? *In Your Healthiest Healthy*, she deals directly with the impact that question had on her and what she did to answer it for herself as well as those around her.

Samantha addresses that and other important issues in a comprehensive, systematic, very readable way. She explains the approaches she took to her new challenge and covers numerous important topics. She reveals the steps she took to improve her nutrition as well as recalibrating her personal health goals. She outlines the program she developed for her physical health with fitness schedules that were realistic and appropriate for her needs, accommodated her treatment, and achieved her goals in a rational, healthy way as well as how she extended that program into her life beyond cancer. She explores the household and personal care items that surround all of us on a daily basis and how they might impact our health, as well as what she did to address them. She shows how she chose her health care team and how she broke her news with family and friends. She delves into the effects that your mindset—mental, emotional, family and social relationships—presents and how that can affect your medical health

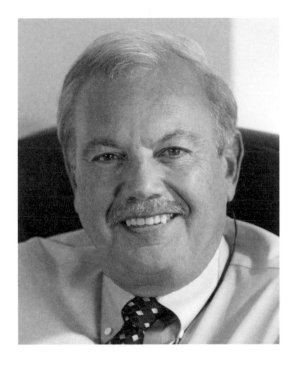

and sense of well being. She does all of this while giving you examples of what worked for her and detailed suggestions of what might work for you as well.

Your Healthiest Healthy shares Samantha's great personal challenge in a way that shows you how, with clear desire and motivation, you can marshal your own inner strength to improve your health and well-being. Her odyssey in answering the big question—"What can I do?"—will give you a road map and game-plan for developing your own approach to a similar challenge.

—Dennis Slamon, MD

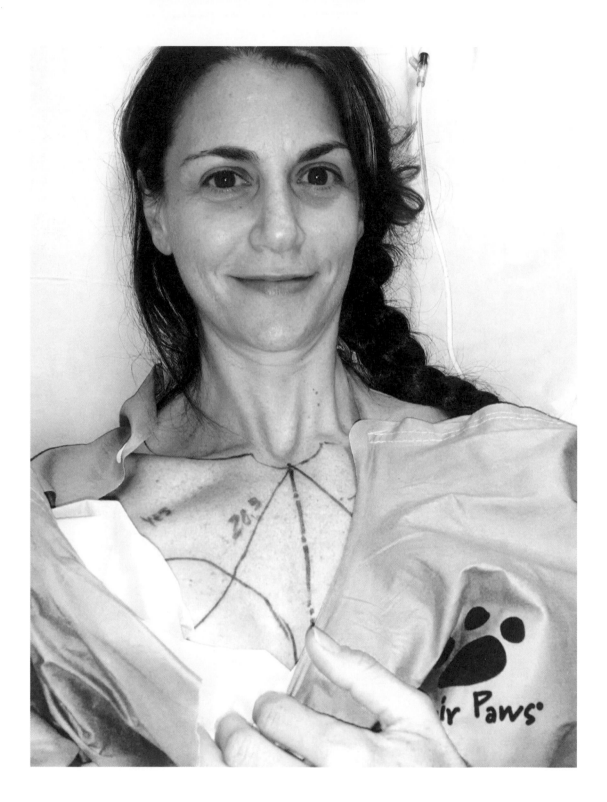

MAKING LEMONADE

My chest still tightens when I talk about that day. It rocked my life—and not in a good way. After my diagnosis and treatment, I obsessed over why this had happened to me and dived headfirst into overhauling my health. I was a fit chick. I didn't eat double-bacon cheeseburgers. I wore sunscreen. I treated cardio like a religion. How did I have cancer? Many people had trudged the same complicated, scary-as-hell road before me. The proliferation of chronic diseases—autoimmune disorders, cancer, diabetes, heart disease—in otherwise "healthy" people—both stunned and scared me. I needed answers.

It took more than two years of poring over books, articles, and websites—plus consultations with nutritionists, internists specializing in integrative medicine, healthy chefs, various oncologists, and other experts—to navigate my way from healthy, to healthier, to my healthiest. There's a lot to process, and, *man*, did I wish someone had given me a road map. That's the reason I'm writing this book, an easy-to-follow guide to taking small, manageable steps to live healthier, cleaner, stronger, and longer and to help you discover the healthiest, happiest, most energized version of yourself.

I always try to set a good example for my two young daughters, so I scheduled my first mammogram right before the big 4–0, when experts recommend that you start getting "the girls" screened. The results came back clear, as expected. I was feeling fit and healthier than ever—but just 11 days later, while changing after a workout class, I found a lump.

D-Day

Somehow I managed to hold it together on the drive from my doctor's office, but now, the second I see him, my legs give out. Michael's loving arms envelop me as I crumble to the ground hysterical. The idea of facing our sweet, innocent girls, who are happily playing at home while waiting for Mommy, destroys me. I can't catch my breath. I can't stop shaking. I have cancer.

Concerned, I hauled ass to my ob-gyn, who said it was nothing, just a normal, glandular effect of getting older. I believed her. Why wouldn't I? Dr. E was my first doctor when I moved to Los Angeles at 23. She was my doc when I lost my virginity at 24. (Spoiler alert: late bloomer!) She coached my husband, Michael, and me through two blissful pregnancies and greeted both of our girls when they came into the world. This woman knew me, and I trusted her.

So I returned to my world of working and workouts, shuttling my kids around and sneaking in some date nights. Yet every time I undressed over the next few weeks, that lump stared me down, taunting me. *What am I? Why am I here?* To make sure I wasn't crazy, I asked my hubby if he could feel it. *Yep.* Could he see it? *Ditto.* So it made sense to have my GP check it out—just to be sure. He also said I had nothing to worry about.

Four months passed, and the lump was still freaking me out. My gut told me to be triple sure, so I scheduled a consult with a surgical oncologist. Two ultrasounds and a needle biopsy later, the oncologist said it didn't seem problematic. *Phew.* But she wasn't sure exactly what it was, so she advised we take it out just to be safe. *Hasta la vista,* lumpy, and *hola* to my first surgery ever.

Back in my surgeon's office, every indication pointed to getting the all clear. *No cancer,* I imagined, *but good for you for being vigilant and an advocate for your own health,* and so on.

Then all of a sudden there it was.

Cancer.

CANCER.

A big, fat, goddamn lemon.

I had stage 1A invasive ductal cancer of the breast: two small tumors, one noninvasive and one smaller, scarier one. As far as diagnoses go, it was a pretty good one. (It's weird to think there's anything "good" about getting cancer, I know!) Treatment would prove complicated

Pulp, Rind, and Then Some

Seriously? Cancer? WTF? I've had more than a week to digest the news, but it still feels like I must be speaking about someone else, not me. I'm young. I eat right, get screened for whatever I should when I should, and I exercise . . . a lot! I'm a friggin' certified personal trainer. I see my doctors for regular checkups. My internist told me he'd be out of business if all his patients were as healthy as I am. This makes no sense.

because the second tumor was invasive, but, hey, it was treatable. The road ahead still felt overwhelming and horrifying.

Surgery options, radiation consults, chemo consults, reconstruction information—spending hours with six of the top surgeons in L.A. made my brain feel like it was about to burst. The first two surgeons told me, hands down, to have a double mastectomy. Cut off the girls, just like that? A third, highly respected surgeon recommended another lumpectomy to remove more tissue, followed by radiation. Either way, it looked like Tamoxifen, an antihormone drug, and I were about to become BFFs to reduce the risk of the cancer returning. Which meant saying hello to early menopause with the possibility of weight gain, night sweats, muscle cramping, hair loss, and vaginal dryness. Hooray!

Michael and I talked about the options for days. We made lists of all of the pros and cons, consulted just about every expert we could find, and flip-flopped . . . a lot. If my cancer was the Super Bowl, we were tied in double overtime.

Here's my first health PSA: Fondle yourself. Seriously, please touch your lady lumps. If you find something, don't wait. Rush to a breast specialist, stat. Getting checked out can be terrifying, but not checking it out is infinitely scarier. Being proactive might have saved my life. In my case, the surgeon who deals with breasts each day made the right call. My other nonspecialist doctors, who are truly fabulous in their own fields, didn't. It's hard not to fault them for thinking it was nothing, but even my lumpectomy surgeon said the *only* person who could have known for *sure* was the pathologist looking at the tissue samples. That's why you gotta be your own health advocate, my friend.

You might be feeling the same way I was in those early days: anxious, confused, and scared as hell about the long road ahead. Feeling desperately lost when it came to my health *sucked*. So I drew on my skills as a seasoned journalist—researching and seeking expert opinions—and called on my background in fitness and nutrition to turn myself from the formerly healthy woman totally stunned by cancer into a stronger, healthier, better-informed survivor and thriver! Along the way, I learned a ton (a whole book full!) about how to forge my own path to better health and happiness, fewer toxins, less stress, and more energy. It's easier said than done—just ask my hubs how many times I wanted to curl up in a ball and, well, bawl—so I'm here to help you figure it out and guide you every step of the way.

During my mastectomy, Dr. Armando Giuliano, my incredibly gifted surgeon, found that the cancer had spread to one of my

Making Lemonade

It's been two weeks of emotional hell. How am I even uttering the words, "I'll be undergoing a double mastectomy"? I can't believe I'm going to lose my breasts. But this surgery will give me the best peace of mind and chance of getting through what hopefully will be my long life without ever having to wear the scarlet letter "C" again. Either I can take it lying down or I can stand up, be strong for myself and our girls, and fight! Boobies, I'm gonna miss ya.

lymph nodes. Hey there, stage 2! Thankfully, he was able to remove it all, so after the mastectomy and two reconstructive surgeries, my oncologists gave me the all clear. Major blessing. My surgery, however, came with some pretty serious aftermath: a newly scarred body, coming to terms with that, zero feeling in my breasts, the back of my arm, and my armpit where they removed several lymph nodes. But if that's the worst of it, count me lucky.

Life gave me a big, fat lemon, which is why, as I lay in a hospital bed, recovering, my hubby reminded me: "Babe, you gotta make lemonade." That little cliché impacted me so much that Michael and I founded a website, GottaMakeLemonade.com, where people dealing with all kinds of life challenges can come together to share their stories, find support, and snag some sweet inspiration in the face of adversity—but more on that later.

Here's where my cancer lemon started to become lemonade. In my new, postcancer reality, reexamining my "healthy" lifestyle became paramount. I had no genetic predisposition for cancer. I went far beyond testing for BRCA mutations; I did a full panel, which tested for any DNA red flags that might spell a health disaster, and came up clean. I've done enough planks and burpees in the last decade to make a boot camp instructor sweat, and my habit of ordering egg-white omelets and cheeseless pizzas (extreme, I admit) prompted almost everyone I knew to give me a Healthiest Eater award. Here I was, the "healthiest" one in the room, but my sports bra had that hot pink "C" emblazoned on it. What was I doing wrong?

Cue a flood of questions. Could the food I scarfed between interviews, TV sets, and my kids' dance practices have created the C-monster? I didn't think so. What about my beloved fitness routine? Did my sweat sessions have the right goals?

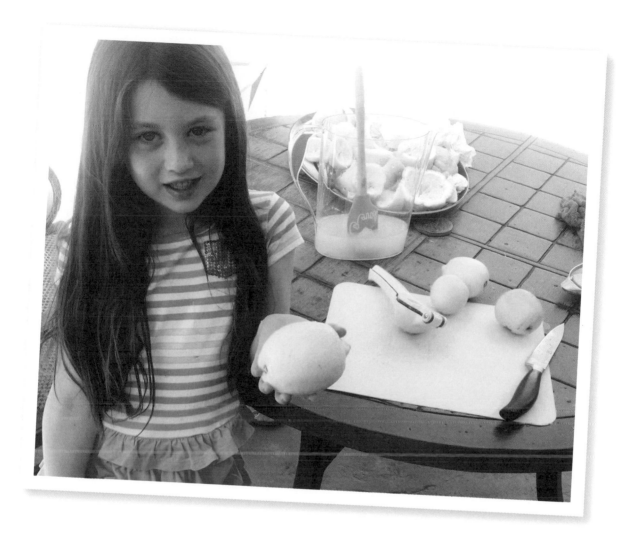

A little research opened the floodgates. Turns out my low-fat, low-cal, diet-foods-by-the-boxload way of eating did need an overhaul. My gym sessions absolutely needed some shaping up. The more I read, the more I felt like Alice falling through the rabbit hole into a Wonderland of research-backed information. I started to wonder about skincare, makeup, and hair products.

What about the scouring, spraying, and sanitizing cleaners we use in our homes? I mean, if the causes weren't inside my body—and we can't control our genetics anyway—could my environment, what I put in, on, and around my body, have invited cancer to come knocking?

You're holding the answer to all that questioning in your hands, my soon-to-be-healthier friend. This book will help guide those who have never had cancer (let's keep it that way), patients and cancer survivors, and those who worry about the other chronic diseases that strike too many of us every year. Take the lessons I've learned and use them to create a healthier, happier life for yourself and your family.

It's not always easy, though. Navigating the labyrinth of sometimes-conflicting health info to figure out what foods are truly healthy, what products are actually toxin-free, and what screenings are absolutely necessary can feel dizzying. This book provides a map out of the labyrinth, one manageable step at a time. Here are the first three steps you need to take:

STEP 1 **RESOLVE TO PURSUE YOUR HEALTHIEST SELF.**

Since you're reading this, you've already done that. Congrats! Ten points for completing step 1!

STEP 2 **EVALUATE WHAT'S WORKING.**

Look at every area of your life: diet, fitness, relationships, and beyond. You'll learn what you need to embrace—green and purple vegetables you like, workouts you love, people who support you, and more. This step also includes being honest with yourself about what's not working and the toxins and negativity you need to ditch.

STEP 3 **TAKE BITE-SIZED ACTION.**

One small step can lead to huge results that will revolutionize your life with hard-core healthiness.

By taking advantage of my experiences and research and the best advice from science and experts, I took something from the cancer monster that it never planned to give: better health and a happier life. Use this book—including the Resources section at the end (page 201)—combine it with your own experiences, and you can create your own action plan for a better, longer, more energized, all-around kick-ass life. I call it your healthiest healthy, and I'm here to help you find it. Hold my hand, laugh at my corny jokes, and let my inner Laker Girl cheer you on. We're in this together. I know you can do it!

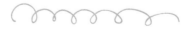

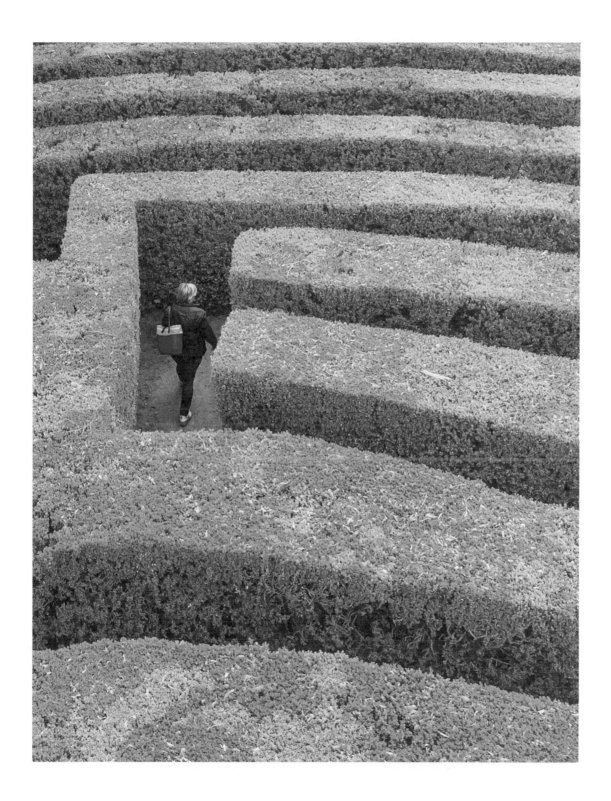

PART ONE

YOUR BODY

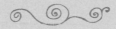

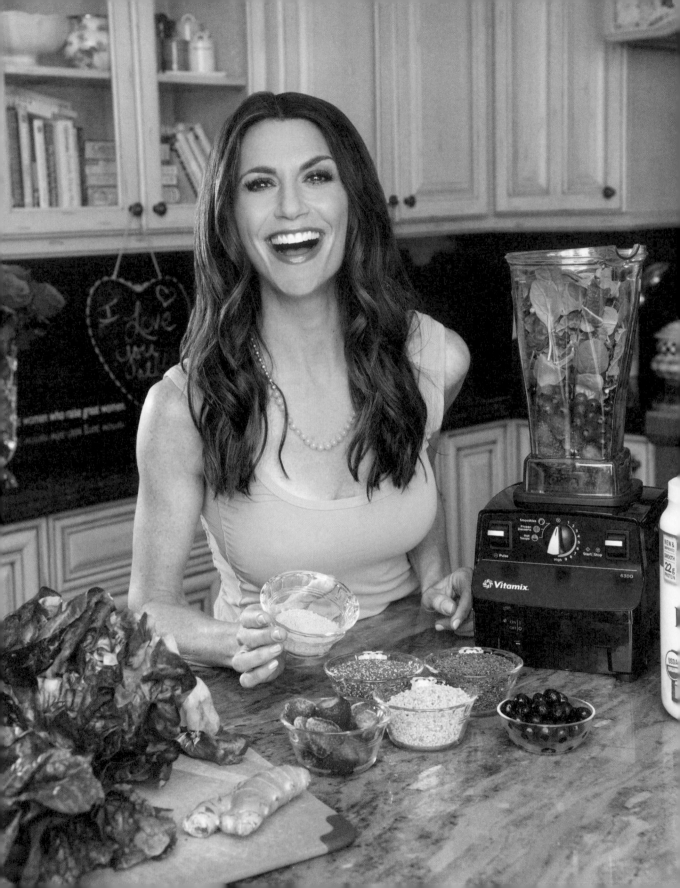

KNOW YOUR NUTRITION

Precancer, eating was about making "healthy" choices so I could rock some serious muscle tone and look hot in a dress (hey, no judgments!). Postcancer, my mindset did a total 180. I booted all my aesthetic concerns and turned up the flame on eating not just for good looks but for good health. No matter how healthy we look, everything we put into our bodies affects our health—down to the cellular level.

On the way to my healthiest healthy, my fat-fearing framework rearranged itself to build a veggie-heavy base, a fiber foundation, and new ways of thinking about carbs, healthy fats, and protein. About freakin' time because studies show that people who eat more vegetables, fab-for-you fats, and other nutrient-rich foods feel better, feel happier, and live longer than those who scarf the same amount of packaged, processed nonfoods.[1]

So get ready for a ride through the tips and treats that helped me reform my inner butter-lover into a better-health advocate. These easy steps will guide you to your healthiest healthy at the grocery store and in your kitchen, one bite at a time.

"HEALTHY" CHOICES

When I was growing up in Minnesota— land of big dairy and red meat—if it mooed, it was food. Mere mention of the word "vegetarian" or "vegan" in Moo-nesota attracted looks of confused scorn, and I was an adventurous carnivore: If it bled, I ate it. I drank half-and-half like skim milk. I used to sneak pats of butter, despite my mom's protests, until I'd finished a whole stick. (I was a pretty sly little devil.) Clearly the concept of health consciousness eluded me as a kid . . . and a teen.

In high school, fast food and soda were my jam, and you always could find two or three pieces of gum stuffed in my mouth. At Northwestern University in Chicago, double-deep-dish pizza was practically a religion. Abstaining from it was a sin, and I became a pious devotee. Add to that my habit of low-fat fro-yo lunches and regular raids into the Delta Gamma kitchen with my sorority sisters to pillage the

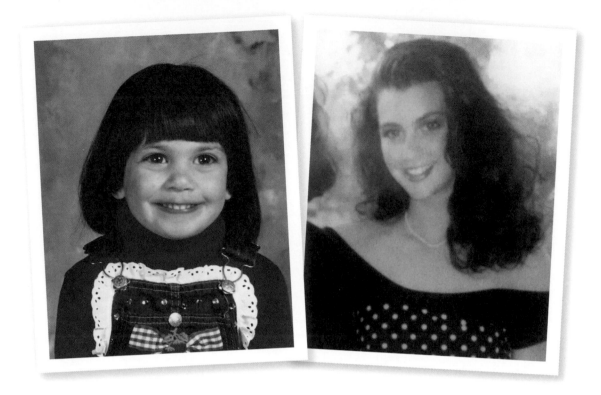

industrial-sized cookie dough supply. Painfully unhealthy, but, hey, college is all about learning, right?

With my diploma came a wizened approach to what I was putting on my plate. My fast-food fetish yielded to a fat-free decree. Then Hollywood called, and the lasso of bad eating habits—the one that ensnares us all when we're trying to balance work and life—got me. Filling my fridge with the makings of healthy, balanced meals wasn't exactly my top priority as a young, broke 20-something in L.A. I worked multiple jobs while trying to high-kick my way through the notoriously impenetrable doors of the entertainment industry. When working as a receptionist, personal assistant, and weekend makeup artist slash manicurist slash food prepper at a kids' tea party place—while juggling auditions—cost is about all that matters, and of course the unhealthy foods, both in the market down the block and at restaurants, were always the least expensive options. The first time my sister, Aimée, came to visit, it shocked her how little food she found in my kitchen. These were my years of food or famine. If the box screamed "low-fat" or "low-cal," it worked for me.

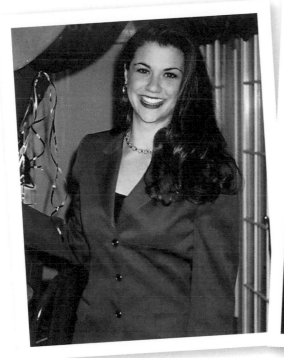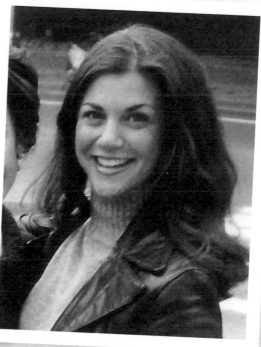

While paying my dues, paycheck to paycheck, my faux-designer purse and I finally landed a steady job at a big-time Hollywood talent management company. Making rent became easier, but that job dealt a blow to my eating habits, which slipped into an office-induced funk: coffee laced with chemical creamers and artificial sweeteners, fast-food takeout, sugar-shock smoothies, and half a box of low-fat vanilla sandwich cookies to get me through the afternoon slump. Compared to my deep-dish days, this counted as "healthy" eating, sure, but, oh baby, did I have a lot to learn.

My first mentor, a wise voice-over actress named Flo, had a day job in the accounting department. She ate to a higher standard of health long before kale and chia started trending. I hadn't even heard of flaxseeds, and she was putting them in her yogurt and sipping green tea before it was cool. She tried to turn me on to (what I thought were) her hippie eating habits, but my low-fat rule convinced me that I had a firm handle on healthy eating.

FROM LOW-FAT TO GOOD HEALTH

For years, scientists told us that low-fat diets held the key to a healthy eating regimen. Now we know that good fats, such as those in avocados and raw almonds, are nutrition powerhouses. So why have we been avoiding fat like the plague for so long?

Fat took a major hit in the 1950s when one pioneering study linked the consumption of saturated fat to heart disease, which is still the leading cause of death in America, according to the Centers for Disease Control and Prevention.[2] That study didn't use a statistically significant sample, however, and it found a link between saturated fats and heart disease only in certain *preselected* countries.[3] Nevertheless, FAT = BAD became the law of the land. Public officials even denied research grants and key posts on expert panels to scientists trying to explore other hypotheses.[4] With today's rigorous scientific standards, no one would take just one flawed study as gospel now.

Also blame the sugar lobby. In the 1960s, the Sugar Research Foundation paid Harvard University scientists big bucks to write a review of studies about sugar, heart disease, and fat—studies that, of course, the Sugar Research Foundation handpicked.[5] One of those paid scientists later became the head of nutrition at the USDA, and he helped draft the dietary guidelines that demonized fat and made sugar look innocuous. Gah!

But not all fats are created equal. More on how to tell the difference between good fats and bad fats later in this chapter.

My big break came at age 29. Fox cast me as host of *The Next Joe Millionaire*, a prime-time show, and then came a gig as the weekend host and full-time correspondent for *Extra*, a syndicated entertainment news show. So did I finally wise up and take Flo's sage advice as I embarked on the first real job of my grown-up career?

Nope. On film and TV sets, the only thing more important than location, trailer sizes, and shooting schedules is the craft-service spread. Cast and crew are only as good as the munchies they eat. Maybe an exaggeration, but you get the idea—food is a big freakin' deal during long shoot days! Cakes, candy, chips, chocolates, cookies, pizza, sliders, and the occasional piece of crudité paraded in front of us daily. As long as I chose the low-fat options, I thought my figure would be fine. For years, these pseudo-healthy choices kept me in a crappy, chemical-filled food rut.

You know how they say everything changes when you have a baby? Well, I thought that meant *after* the little nugget pops out. In my case, everything changed before she was born—and not just my hips widening! For years, my fitness regimen kept me in pretty good shape, and, in my mind, as long as the pounds stayed off, I was making healthy choices. But when I realized that I was creating another human being, it finally dawned on me that a lot of my food choices—salads with sugar-saturated dressings, highly processed whole wheat breads, nonorganic chicken breasts—were lacking in nutrients at best and packed with chemicals at worst. Ensuring that my growing fetus was absorbing something better than sandwich cookies opened the door to my healthier healthy.

At that point, I was the Girl Who Skipped Breakfast, running on heavily sweetened coffee and fructose-filled yogurt until 11 a.m., at which point I gobbled several slices of turkey bacon. (Confession: My fantastic *E! News* coworkers didn't appreciate my toaster-oven-cured meat stinking up the studio kitchen every day. Sorry, guys!)

The most helpful recommendations then came from my friend Christine Avanti-Fischer, a certified nutritionist, fitness expert, and author of *Skinny Chicks Eat Real Food*. She taught me the importance of maintaining an even-keel metabolism with balanced meals, every three to four hours, that contained protein, carbohydrates, and healthy fats. That was the first time anyone ever told me I was *supposed* to eat fat. Who knew?

She was so right. Studies show that grabbing a morning meal helps curb hunger throughout the day, lowers your risk of diabetes and heart disease, and can help whittle your waistline. Several studies with kids also show that eating breakfast results in a brain boost.[6] So breakfast became my buddy. Focusing on eating a healthy balance of nutrients daily—including the formerly forbidden F-word—helped boost my energy and stamina, and it made my pregnancy go more smoothly. Still, I had no clue how much further down the path to feeling amazing I had to go.

Years later, after recovering from my mastectomy, I immediately went to see an integrative specialist, an MD who uses a battery of traditional and nontraditional health techniques. She handed me two books. One was thicker than a dictionary, weighed as much as my three-year-old, and looked like it would put me to sleep before it put me on the path to better eating. The second

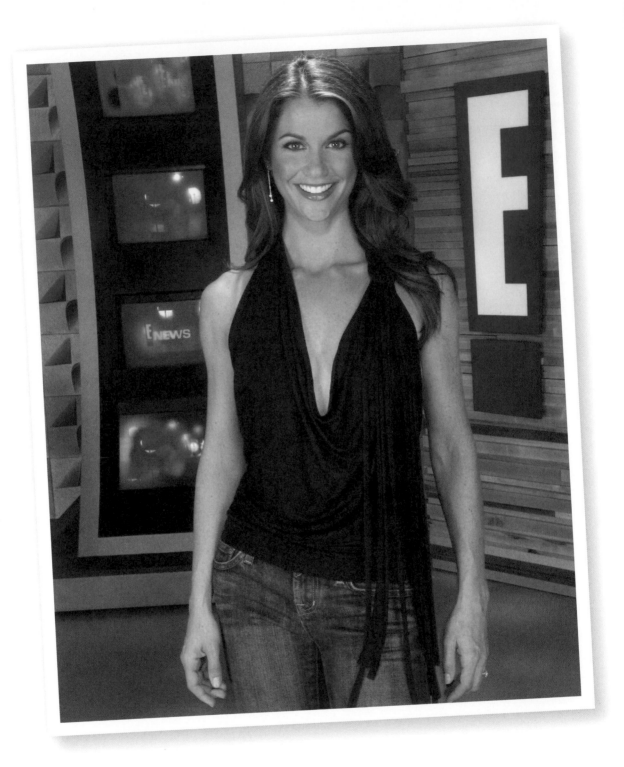

YOUR HEALTHIEST HEALTHY

book, *Eat to Lose, Eat to Win* by Rachel Beller, RDN, looked more fun and strangely familiar. Turns out another copy was collecting dust (sorry, Rachel) somewhere on my desk at home. I digested her totally doable nutrition revolution so quickly and so well that I reached out to work with her directly. Since then, she's created an even more updated nutritional program, called PowerPerks, aimed at breast cancer prevention.

Hiring a nutritionist to help you overhaul your pantry isn't an option for everyone, but that's why I'm here to help. You and I are on this journey together, my soon-to-be healthier friend—including meal fails and moments of frustration so strong you want to scarf down a box of Girl Scout cookies. It's all part of the path to finding your healthiest healthy.

HEALTHY HACK

You don't have to give up every joy in life. I mean, come on, you gotta bend the rules for those adorable Girl Scouts once a year! It's all about finding the right balance between reducing nutrient-deficient foods and upping the healthful ones so you can live a more energized, healthful life. My abiding love for the occasional Thin Mint helps make living my healthiest life worth it. You should enjoy your eating habits!

KEEP A FOOD JOURNAL

Before you embark on your own nutrition revolution, you gotta know where you're starting, and that means keeping a detailed food journal. For six weeks, I want you to track every mouthful. Write down exactly what you eat for breakfast, lunch, dinner, and snacks. Don't forget to record what liquids you drink, too, including water. Also consider recording portion size and what time you ate or drank each item. What you find might surprise you, and it might help you make better choices in the future.

HEALTHY HACK

Keep portion size in mind when tracking your food. If you down a whole bag of baked chips at your desk in one day, that's probably closer to three servings. Check the label (more on that later). Honesty pays off big-time when you're figuring out which areas you need to improve. Sometimes it hurts to write it down, but if you fib, you're only keeping yourself from success.

Here's what my food journal looked like as I moved from healthy(ish), to healthier, to healthiest.

MORNING MEAL

HEALTHY(ISH)

* 1 cup coffee with fat-free half-n-half and 2 packets Splenda
* 1 banana
* Weekend: 1 cinnamon raisin bagel with cream cheese, 3 egg whites scrambled with veggies, 1 cup sliced fruit, and 1 cup store-bought orange juice

HEALTHIER

* 1 blueberry nonfat Greek yogurt with crushed granola topping
* 1 cup fresh-squeezed orange juice
* 1 banana
* Weekend: 1 scooped-out whole wheat bagel with cream cheese and jelly, 3 egg whites scrambled with veggies, 2 cups sliced fruit, 1 cup fresh-squeezed orange juice

♡ HEALTHIEST ♡

* 3¾ cups smoothie with organic dark leafy greens, berries, plant-based protein powder, matcha green tea powder, greens powder, ginger, bee pollen, chia, and flaxseeds. Check out the recipe on page 25!

MIDDAY MEAL #1

HEALTHY(ISH)

* 7 slices turkey bacon, 1 cup sucrose-filled light yogurt
* 8 ounces fresh-squeezed orange juice

HEALTHIER

* sliced turkey sandwich on whole wheat bread with lettuce, roasted red peppers, cucumbers, and honey mustard
* carrots and hummus

♡ HEALTHIEST ♡

* 1 huge chopped salad with organic romaine lettuce, purple cabbage, cherry tomatoes, cucumbers, broccoli, red bell peppers, carrots, celery, avocado, lentils, and garbanzo beans tossed with balsamic vinegar, lemon pepper, turmeric, and a light drizzle of extra virgin olive oil.
* 2 handfuls bean & rice nacho chips

MIDDAY MEAL #2

HEALTHY(ISH)

* 3¾ cups smoothie made with vanilla yogurt, orange juice, frozen berries and banana, and ice
* 1 sleeve Thin Mint cookies

HEALTHIER

* 1 apple with 1–2 tablespoons reduced-fat big brand peanut butter

♡ HEALTHIEST ♡

* 1 organic apple with almond butter or cucumbers, carrots, and celery with hummus

DINNER

HEALTHY(ISH)

* Parmesan chicken arrabiata, pasta with sautéed veggies
* ice cream or microwave popcorn, plus candy, candy, candy

HEALTHIER

* whole wheat pasta with chicken breast, broccoli, roasted red peppers, and asparagus
* ice cream or 1 big handful dark chocolate raisins

♡ HEALTHIEST ♡

* 1 black bean burger topped with guac and tomatoes on sprouted whole grain bun. Check out the recipe on page 32.
* Heaps of roasted organic veggies (broccoli, Brussels sprouts, carrots) or cauliflower rice
* 2–4 squares 73 percent cacao dark chocolate

As you can see, my healthy(ish) entries seriously lacked anything green and were swimming in sugar. They weren't *totally* unhealthy, but they had lots of room for improvement. When I found my healthier healthy, breakfast became a real meal, and whole grains replaced starchy carbs. A small, easy step with a big impact! But it still was lacking significantly in green goodness and other nutrient-dense foods. In my healthiest healthy, organic veggies fill my plate or cup at every meal, healthy fats abound, beans and nuts rule my recipes, power-boosters such as ginger and turmeric work their magic daily, and sugar stays on the bench.

This isn't about cleaning out your fridge and switching to kale and wheatgrass overnight. That would have scared the bejeezus out of me (although, confession: I have become a bit of a kale fangirl). Rachel carefully reviewed my food journal to see where I could make small, relatively painless nutrition tweaks.

That's where it starts for you, too. Small steps lead to big results. The nutrition knowledge that follows will empower you to make simple, gradual changes. Every one, even the teeny ones, will help you achieve better overall health. If you can make one small change at every meal, you're killing it! The only way to fail is not to try. Read on, pick a couple of nuggets that seem easy, and try them out. When they become part of your daily diet, come back for more. Little by little, you'll go a long way, baby!

Grab that food journal and let's do this.

NUTRITION LABEL KNOW-HOW

A big part of upping your nutrition knowledge requires reading the nutrition label the right way. Easier said than done. Obsessing over ingredients seems like a big ask when you're rushing through the grocery store, but it's worth it. Women who read labels have a BMI that's 1.49 points lower than those who don't, according to a 2012 study that looked at the effects of nutrition labels on obesity.[7] Extra poundage can lead to chronic diseases, so that's a big deal.[8]

Case in point: My family's not-so-smart love of a certain smart cereal. For years, I thought I was being such a conscientious mommy by giving my hubby and kids a good start every morning. Smart is right there in the name! The copy on the box says it contains whole grains, so how could that not be an intelligent choice? But marketing guys are sneaky. A closer look at the label revealed that the cereal had a stupid finish. Here's what to look for on a nutrition label to make sure you're fueling your bod with the right stuff.

Nutrition Facts

8 servings per container

Serving size   **2/3 cup (55g)**

Amount per serving

Calories   230

	% Daily Value*
Total Fat 8g	**10%**
Saturated Fat 1g	**5%**
Trans Fat 0g	
Cholesterol 0mg	**0%**
Sodium 160mg	**7%**
Total Carbohydrate 37g	**13%**
Dietary Fiber 4g	**14%**
Total Sugars 12g	
Includes 10g Added Sugars	**20%**
Protein 3g	
Vitamin D 2mcg	10%
Calcium 260mg	20%
Iron 8mg	45%
Potassium 235mg	6%

* The % Daily Value (DV) tells you how much a nutrient in a serving of food contributes to a daily diet. 2,000 calories a day is used for general nutrition advice.

Go Beyond Calorie Count

It's tempting to check for calories and then call it a day, but the label contains a lot of important info. We're focusing on essential nutrients here, not calories. The government recommends that the average moderately active woman—meaning you work out a couple of times a week and hit your step goal during the day—should eat between 2,000 and 2,200 calories per day to maintain a healthy weight.[9] That may be too many calories for some and not enough for active chiquitas, so know your body and adjust accordingly.

Not All Fats Are Created Equal

When it comes to trans fats, anything higher than zero is unacceptable. Drop it and walk away. For saturated fats—which increase your levels of bad cholesterol and your risk of heart disease—total consumption shouldn't exceed 6 percent of your total calorie intake, according to the American Heart Association.[10] That means no more than 13 grams of sat fat per day. Do fewer if you can!

Fiber

Lots of nutrition lists feature fiber additives. These fillers technically count as fiber but don't deliver the nutritional benefits of the natural stuff. Real fiber comes only from whole grains, beans, fruit, and veggies. Keep that in mind when tallying your daily fiber intake. Aim for 30 or more grams per day.

Sneaky Sugars

The sugar industry has found ways of sneaking the sweet stuff into everything. Even foods you don't think of as sweet, such as bread or tomato sauce, can have a *ton* of added sugars. Fruits, for example, have lots of natural sugars, which isn't necessarily bad. It's the *added* sugars that are a killer. Look out for these bad boys and make sure that no more than 10 percent of your calories come from added sugars.[11]

Protein

The more protein in your morning meal, the better. Research shows that people who eat 35 grams of protein at breakfast feel less hungry throughout the day and also experience a brain boost that helps control appetite.[12] But try not to get it from meat or dairy. Plant-based proteins are best (more on that in a bit).

Understand the Ingredients

Pay close attention to the first three ingredients. What goes into packaged food is listed by weight, so you're getting the most of the first item, and the last item might be present only in trace amounts. In the case of my not-so-smart cereal, the first ingredient is rice. That's healthier than some ingredients in other cereals, sure, but it's not great. When rice hits your stomach, your body turns it into sugar in a snap.[13] Second ingredient: whole grain wheat, which is always a solid staple, so good there. Third ingredient: sugar, which also shows up fifth, sixth, and tenth as brown

rice syrup, corn syrup, and honey. Nope. That cereal had to go. When it did, my hubby dropped pounds like nobody's biz, and his newfound green smoothies make him more energized. (See, wifey's nagging isn't *always* a bad thing!) If you're not sure what something is, look it up! Again, you might be surprised at what you find.

YOUR COMPLETE PANTRY-TO-PLATE MAKEOVER

Now that you know how to read a nutrition label effectively, you need to look at what's in your kitchen. Get rid of the chemical-filled nonfoods and focus on the good stuff. Don't do it all at once, though. Take it step by step and incorporate it organically into your daily routine.

STEP 1 Slash the Sugar.

My food journal revealed a major issue: my sweet tooth. Soda fell by the wayside years ago, but my love affair with candy was a battle. Rachel Beller, my nutritionist, told me that sugar invaded every meal, but what did she mean?

Added sugars hide everywhere: "healthy" yogurt, ketchup, orange juice, pizza sauce, protein bars, salad dressing, and even freakin' whole wheat bread. My morning blueberry yogurt topped with a crumbled granola bar sounded healthy, but here's where nutrition label know-how matters. That yogurt had *16 grams* of sugar per serving! Better to go with the naturally low-sugar plain version and add fresh blueberries. If it needs a little lick of sweetness, drizzle a little raw honey on it. I know, honey is sugar, but it's *natural* sugar, not chemically created, and you can control how much you add. I started with one tablespoon every morning and weaned myself down to just one teaspoon or less. Take that, sweet tooth!

Since my diagnosis, I've heard time and again that sugar feeds cancer. I've asked my oncologists about it, and they disagree. They say that no conclusive studies prove this theory. But we know that sugar doesn't do a body good. Tons of studies show that letting your sweet tooth call the shots can up your risk of developing diabetes and dying of heart disease.[14]

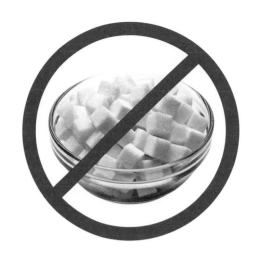

HEALTHY HACK

The sugar industry camouflages its goodies really well. They have dozens of different names for their sweet stuff. Cane syrup, dextrose, fruit juice concentrate, galactose, maltodextrin, maltose, sucrose, barley malt, or treacle on an ingredients list means sugar. Bench those bad boys!

STEP 2 **Unleash Your Inner Veggie.** Raw veggies, especially those with green or purple hues, have hugely powerful anticancer, anti-inflammatory, and anti–chronic disease properties.[15] Research shows that crunching on copious amounts of cruciferous and leafy veggies fuels us with optimism, slims us down, boosts our longevity, and most importantly lessens our risk of developing cancer, heart disease, and other chronic conditions.[16]

If, as mine did, your plate typically features a big hunk of animal protein with a small serving of veggies and carbs, flip those proportions. Veggies should fill half a perfect plate. Yes, at least *half.* Pack the rest of it with protein, ideally plant-based (beans and legumes), good carbs (such as yams or brown rice), and a dab of healthy fat.

SMOOTHIE CENTRAL

With the right recipe, smoothies offer a yummy way to hit your veggie quota. Before you balk at veggies for breakfast, hear me out. In one delicious drink, you can get a serious serving of fiber, nutrient-dense goodness, omega-3s, kick-ass antioxidants, and essential vitamins and minerals—that's one small sip for your morning meal and one giant slurp on the road to your healthiest healthy. Starting your day with veggies often makes you crave more throughout the day. Totally true for me, and that's a good craving to indulge.

Figuring out how to get all those goodies into something that tastes, well, *tasty* comes down to practice. Sip-sized steps are your friend here. Loading your blender with yogurt, fruit, and ice may taste like a dream, and, yeah, it can help you hop on the smoothie train, but work on cutting the sugar and upping the nutrients. Here are some easy tweaks to get even the pickiest smoothie newbie on board:

* Add a heaping spoonful of chia seeds. It won't change the flavor, but it boosts the fiber and healthy fat content.
* Ditch the sugary yogurt or OJ and sub in almond milk or water. For a creamier version, try cashew milk.

To get a hefty serving of protein into your morning meal without leaning too much on dairy, try a heaping spoonful of plant-based protein powder. My fave brands are Vega, Sunwarrior, and especially Garden of Life, which mixes with ease and tastes oh-so-delicious.

Now for the big guns, those veggies. The baby-step solution? Spinach. It has a mild taste while packing tons of vitamins and minerals, such as iron; vitamins A, C, and K; folate; and potassium. Eventually you won't even notice the spinach. When you've mastered that hack, go wild and toss in some kale or even collard greens. They're not just for sautéing anymore!

HEALTHY HACK

A little pineapple helps mask kale's bitter taste. Also tap your inner massage therapist and give your kale a good knead before blending, which helps break up that tough texture and cuts the bitterness. Sounds weird, but it totally works.

For the recipes that follow, place all ingredients in a blender and blend until smooth.

Banana Cinnamon Date Smoothie

YIELD **1½–2 cups**   PREP TIME **5 minutes**

* 8–10 ounces unsweetened cashew milk (or other nut milk)
* 1½ cups ice
* 1 frozen banana
* 1 or 2 pitted Medjool dates
* ½–¾ cup rolled oats
* 1 tablespoon chia seeds
* ½ teaspoon matcha green tea powder
* Ceylon cinnamon to taste
* healthy bonus: 1 handful kale or spinach

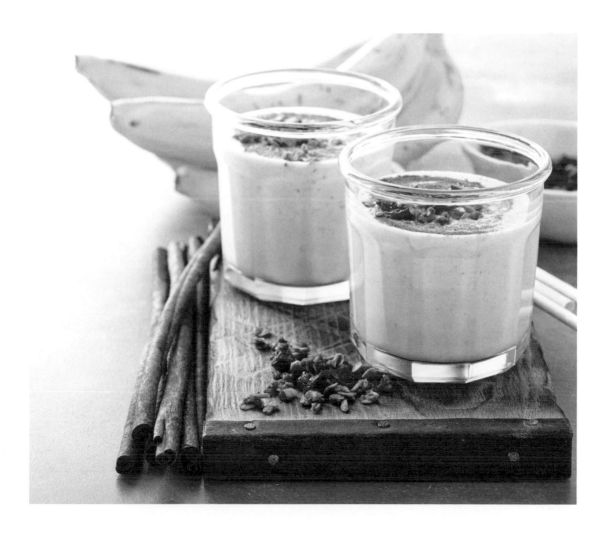

Chocolate Peanut Butter Banana Smoothie

YIELD **1½–2 cups** PREP TIME **5 minutes**

* 8–10 ounces unsweetened vanilla almond, cashew, or soy milk
* 1½ cups ice
* 2 frozen bananas
* 1 scoop chocolate protein powder
* 1 tablespoon natural peanut butter
* ¾ tablespoon raw cacao nibs
* healthy bonus: 1 tablespoon chia or flaxseeds

Samantha's Smoothie

YIELD **5 cups** PREP TIME **15 minutes**

* 10–14 ounces filtered water
* 2 handfuls spinach
* 1 handful kale
* 3–4 leaves collard greens (optional, in lieu of kale)
* 1½–2 cups frozen strawberries
* 1–1½ cups frozen blueberries
* 1–1½ scoops plant-based vanilla protein powder
* 1 scoop greens powder
* 1–1½ teaspoons matcha green tea powder
* 1–2 tablespoons chia seeds
* 1 tablespoon flaxseeds
* 1½ inches gingerroot, peeled

This recipe makes a lot, and I often save half of it for a midmorning snack. Choose organic produce whenever possible.

What healthy smoothies do you like? Share with me on social media! I'm here to answer your questions, cheer you on, and swap recipes. My coordinates are at the end of my author bio at the back of the book.

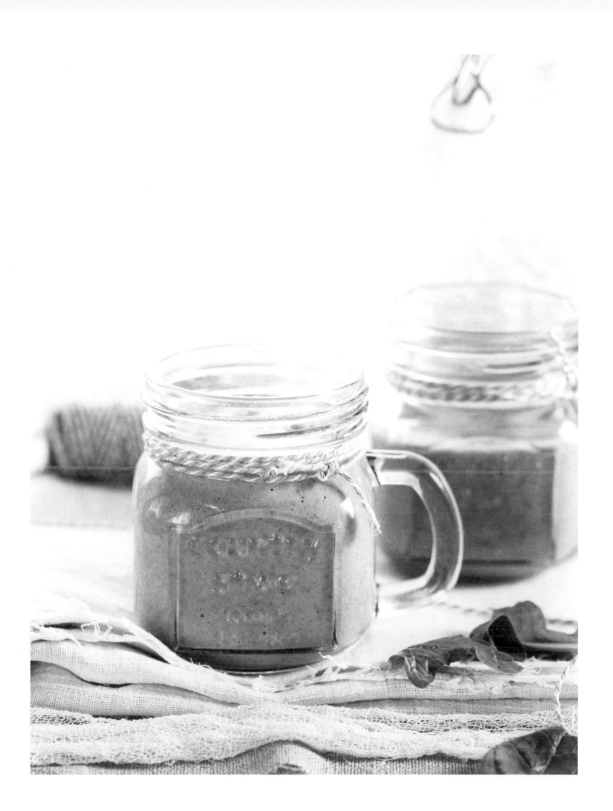

TRAIN YOUR TASTE BUDS

Know how you can train your pet? Use small, gradual steps and reward good behavior. Same works for your hubby—love you, honey!—and your taste buds. How cool is that? According to the experts, it can take as few as three days to nix a bad habit and start a healthier craving.[17] Turn your buds into buddies like this:

* **Consistency is key.** Try it again and again . . . and *again*.
* **Easy does it.** One thing at a time. Don't overwhelm your palate with a full-on assault.
* **Buddy up.** Add your healthy new food to something you know you enjoy. Add kale to your favorite smoothie recipe or snack on carrots dipped in ranch dressing before learning to love them solo. (It worked for my kiddos, too.)
* **Knowledge is crucial.** When you know the nutritional and health bennies, you have more motivation to stick with it.

HEALTHY HACK

If you always eat a meaty sandwich for lunch, transition slowly. Add the same ingredients to a bed of lettuce instead of bread and gradually swap the meat for protein-packed beans.

One of the easiest places to hit your veggie quota is in a big ol' salad for lunch. At the beginning of the week, I chop up my green goods and dish it out daily in big portions. My daily salad is ridiculously huge. Just beware that all salads aren't healthy by definition. Adding croutons, cheese, and heavy dressing increases your unhealthy fats and sugars fast.

This switch to a veggie-heavy lifestyle has given me tremendous energy, and all it took was a few small steps—a green smoothie here, a veggie-packed salad there. Start with two veggie-based meals a week. Give it a month, see how you feel, then up the veggie ante!

Instead of store-bought dressing—which is packed with sugar, laden with chemicals, and expensive—make your own in a flash: a squeeze of fresh lemon juice, a dribble of extra virgin olive oil, a dash of balsamic vinegar, maybe some fresh minced garlic, and a sprinkle of lemon pepper to top it all off. Throw some turmeric on top for anti-oxidant bonus points!

STEP 3 **Fill Up with Fiber.**
Fiber helps lower blood sugar levels, keeps the scale from hitting the OMG zone, and makes your poops as regular as your morning alarm.[18] The government officially recommends 25 grams of fiber per day, but many health experts think that's not enough.[19] To make sure I got the Rachel-recommended 30–35 grams of fiber per day, she suggested front-loading in the morning with heavy-hitters such as chia seeds, kale, and blueberries, aiming for about 15 grams total. In your quest for crunch, look for labels that feature simple ingredients, such as wheat germ, that you can pronounce and that don't come from a lab.

One of my favorite ways to flex the fiber in my diet is through flax, sesame, and chia seeds, which helped me ditch the crunchy, sugary granola topping for breakfast. They're also kick-ass cancer fighters—especially breast cancer. Compounds in these teeny body boosters bind to estrogen receptors and help prevent the cancer-feeding effects that estrogen can have on breast tissue.[20] In other words, they're big antioxidant boosters, so load up on 'em.

After a week of putting Rachel's fiber recs into practice, not only was I still standing, but no more wrestling with the growling beast in my stomach as the clock slowly ticked to lunchtime. Try it for a week and see if you feel fuller and more energetic, too!

HEALTHY HACK

Watch out for fiber additives. Inulin, chic-ory root, and polydextrose technically count as fiber, but they're not as nutritious as the natural fiber in whole grains, seeds, fruits, and veggies.

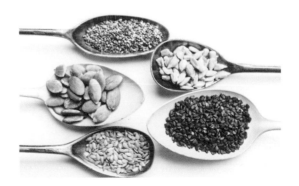

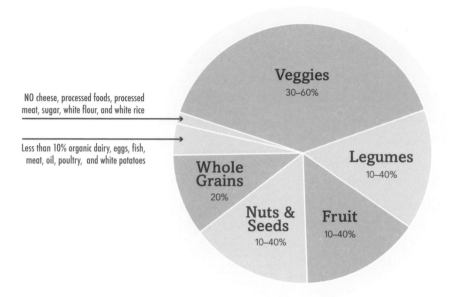

NO cheese, processed foods, processed meat, sugar, white flour, and white rice

Less than 10% organic dairy, eggs, fish, meat, oil, poultry, and white potatoes

Veggies
30–60%

Legumes
10–40%

Whole Grains
20%

Nuts & Seeds
10–40%

Fruit
10–40%

STEP 4 **Peruse New Protein.**
Protein is your body's building block. It keeps your cells functioning and is essential for healthy hair, skin, and bones.[21] But not all protein is created equal.

The more researchers learn about meat, the bleaker it looks for cow-chowing. In 2015, the World Health Organization officially recognized that processed meats, such as sausage and my beloved toaster-oven turkey bacon, increase your risk for cancer. Red meat, such as beef and lamb, *probably* ups your cancer risk.[22] Those findings form just part of a huge body of research illuminating the ills of animal protein. *The China Study*, a book based on a massive nutritional study started in the

1980s by biochemist T. Colin Campbell, found that the closer people come to a plant-based diet, the lower their risk of chronic diseases.[23] So get your sweet self to the garden, girl!

Eat to Live by Dr. Joel Fuhrman, along with Rachel's advice and *The China Study*, has shaped my nutrition revolution. "All animal products, including meat, fish, and dairy, are low (or completely lacking) in the nutrients that protect us against cancer and heart attacks," Dr. Fuhrman writes. "Animal products are rich in substances that scientific investigations have shown to be associated with the incidence of cancer and heart disease: saturated fat, cholesterol, and arachidonic acid."[24]

No need to start hoarding turkey burgers. You don't have to become a vegetarian or a vegan to reach your healthiest healthy. In a recent study, researchers at Harvard University found that replacing meat with plant-based protein at even one meal a week lowered the risk of heart disease, diabetes, and obesity.[25] Start slow and keep going.

That said, some exceptions do apply. "While some animal products are low in nutrients that may provide protection from cancer, others contain nutrients that may provide some benefits, such as wild salmon," Rachel says. "Omega-3 fatty acids found in fish have the ability to fight pro-inflammatory enzymes that promote breast cancer. They also can protect against heart disease and rheumatoid arthritis, reduce inflammation, enhance cognitive function, and nourish the skin." She took one look at my habit of gobbling poultry at 10 to 12 meals a week and gave me a new goal: Limit my fowl intake to just 2 or 3 meals a week, filling the gaps with 2 to 3 servings of low-mercury fish for those omega-3s and the rest

with vegetarian options, such as beans, organic sprouted tofu, and tempeh (more like "temp-blech" in my opinion).

What was a meat-loving girl to do? Yep, that's right, small steps. Chickpeas already occupied some real estate in my pantry, so they began playing a bigger role in my salads. Munch 'em raw or toss them with a little extra-virgin olive oil and roast them in the oven for a fantastic crunchy alternative to croutons. If you're searching for other places to add more legumes—think lentils and white beans—soups and chilis are a great place to start.

Amazingly, poultry petered out after a year of slow changes and now appears on my plate only occasionally. Go full veggie or vegan *only* if you're into it and can count whole foods and plant-based nutrients as the staples of your meals; if not, mind your meat consumption.

HEALTHY HACK

Another easy protein swap is lentil or black bean pasta. Tolerant makes an awesome, protein-packed one that turns carby dishes into big, veggie-friendly providers of protein and fiber. If you're gaga for garbanzos, try Banza's chickpea pasta.

HEALTHY OFFICE LUNCHES

Rushed lunch breaks and subpar cafeteria options don't jive with eating for your healthiest self. Thankfully, brown-bagging it these days doesn't mean eating the sad-sack lunch of your childhood memories. Here are some of my favorite healthy homemade meals that will make you the envy of the office.

Black Bean Burgers

YIELD **6 patties**   PREP TIME **20 minutes**   COOK TIME **25 minutes**   TOTAL TIME **45 minutes**

* 1 sweet potato, peeled and chopped
* 1 pinch Himalayan or sea salt
* 2 tablespoons avocado oil
* ½ cup finely diced onion
* 1 (16-ounce) can black beans
* 1 cup cooked brown rice
* ⅛ cup panko bread crumbs
* 2 cloves garlic, minced
* ½ tablespoon ground cumin
* 1 teaspoon chili powder
* 1 teaspoon Himalayan or sea salt
* 3 tablespoons tamari
* 2 teaspoons vegan Worcestershire sauce
* extra-virgin olive oil

1. Preheat the oven to 425°F.

2. Mix sweet potato, pinch of salt, and 1 tablespoon avocado oil in a heat-proof dish and roast 20–25 minutes, until sweet potatoes are tender.

3. In a small sauté pan, brown the onion on medium heat with 1 tablespoon avocado oil.

4. In a food processor, combine all the rest of the ingredients, except for the olive oil, with the sweet potato and onion mixture and pulse. Be careful not to overmix. Let the mixture cool in the fridge for about an hour, then form into 6 (6-ounce) patties.

5. Thinly coat the burgers on both sides with olive oil and brown them in a cast-iron skillet or sauté pan on medium-high heat.

6. Serve on sprouted whole grain buns topped with guacamole, fresh tomatoes, or salsa.

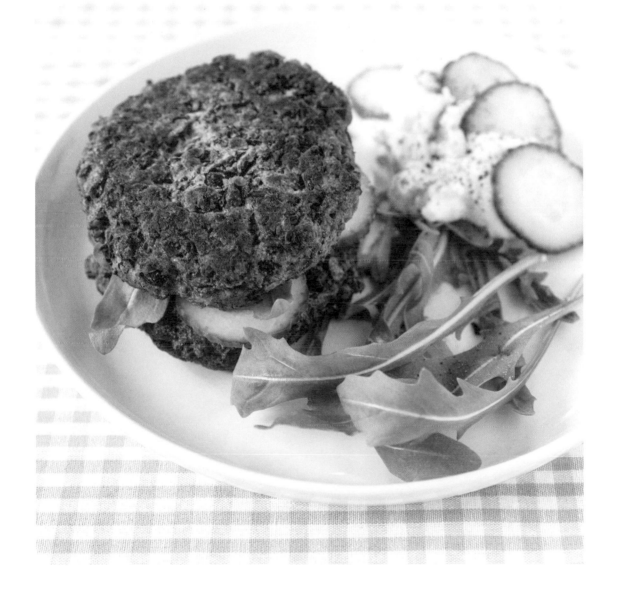

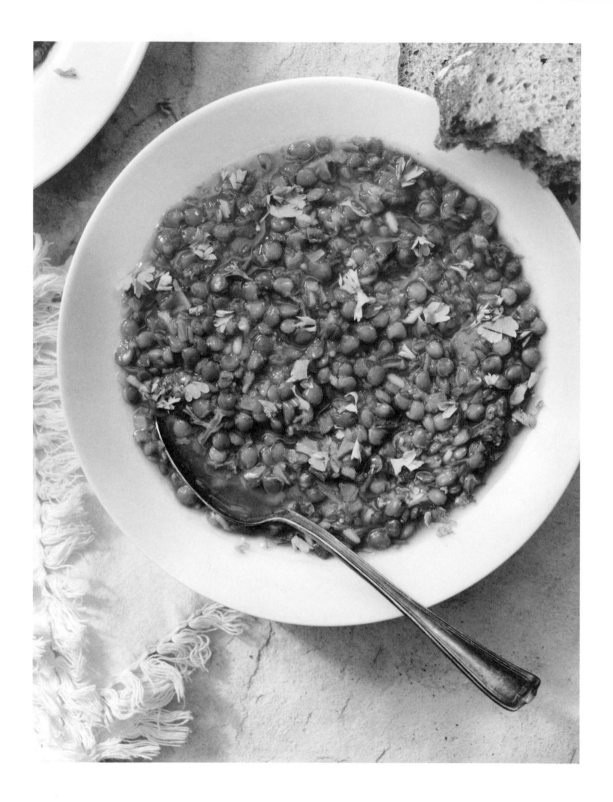

YOUR HEALTHIEST HEALTHY

Lentil Soup

YIELD **4 servings**   PREP TIME **40 minutes**   COOK TIME **30 minutes**   TOTAL TIME **1 hour 10 minutes**

* 1 cup lentils
* 1 large yellow onion, diced
* 1 cup carrots, diced
* ¾ cup celery, chopped
* 2 tablespoons extra-virgin olive oil
* 1 tablespoon minced garlic
* ½ teaspoon thyme
* 1 teaspoon pink Himalayan salt
* ¼ teaspoon fresh ground black pepper, or to taste
* 6 cups low-sodium vegetable broth
* 2 tablespoons tomato paste
* 1 teaspoon red wine vinegar
* chopped parsley or scallions, to taste, as garnish

1. Using precooked lentils will cut your prep time in half. If you're using dry lentils, rinse them thoroughly and place them in a heatproof bowl.

2. Boil enough water to cover the lentils, pour the water over the lentils, and let them soak for 20 minutes. Then drain the water.

3. Sauté onion, carrots, and celery in the olive oil until tender, for about 10 minutes. Add the garlic, thyme, salt, and pepper.

4. In a food processor or a high-speed blender, blend two-thirds of the lentils.

5. Combine blended lentils, the remaining whole lentils, the vegetable broth, tomato paste, and sautéed veggies in a pot over medium-high heat. Bring to a boil, then reduce heat and simmer until the whole lentils become tender, about 30 minutes.

6. Remove from heat. Place half the soup mixture in a food processor and pulse gently, then put it back in the pot to mix together. Stir in the vinegar, and garnish with parsley or scallions.

Chickpea Salad

YIELD **4 servings**   PREP TIME **1 hour 15 minutes**

* 3 cups chickpeas (no added salt)
* 1 medium stalk celery, chopped
* 1–2 dill pickles, finely chopped
* 2 tablespoons vegan mayo or half an avocado
* 1½ teaspoons tamari or low-sodium soy sauce
* 1 tablespoon pickle juice or lime juice
* Himalayan or sea salt and fresh ground pepper, to taste
* 3–4 romaine leaves or collard green wraps

1. Mash chickpeas with a fork until smushed but not totally smooth.

2. Add all the remaining ingredients except for the lettuce or collard greens, mix, and chill in the fridge for about 1 hour.

3. Serve in romaine leaves or collard green wraps.

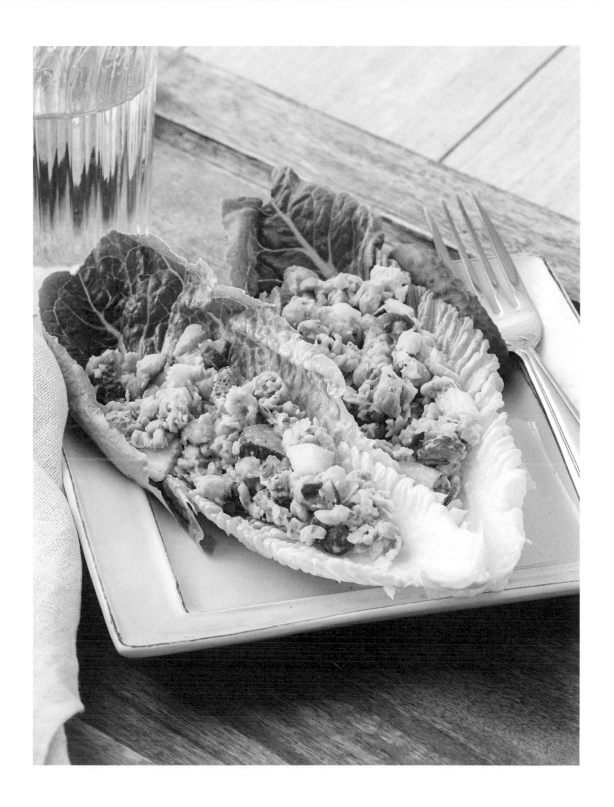

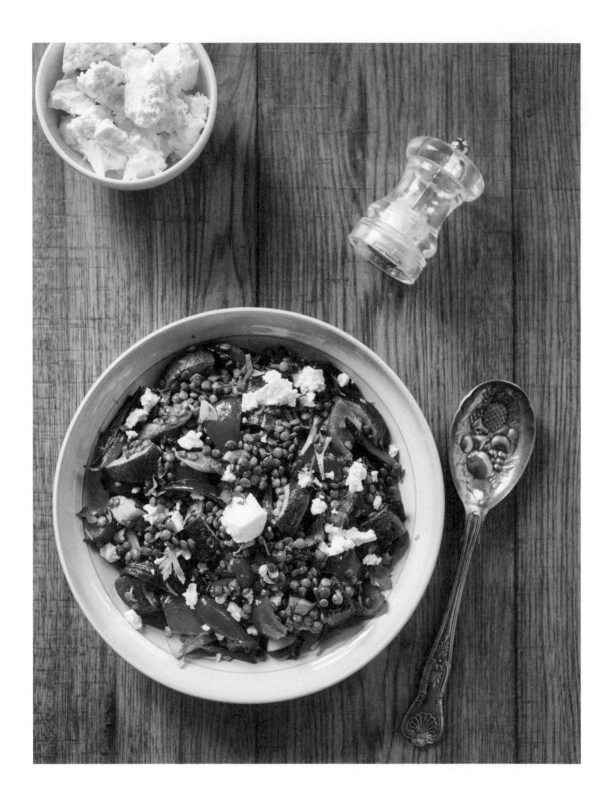

YOUR HEALTHIEST HEALTHY

Lentil Chopped Salad

YIELD **2 servings**   PREP TIME **45 minutes**

Customize this recipe with your favorite healthiest healthy veggies for maximum enjoyment and variety, and this rainbow of goodness will look mighty pretty on Instagram.

* 4 cups chopped greens
* 1 cup chopped purple cabbage
* 2–3 cups chopped organic veggies of your choice (broccoli, celery, carrots, red bell peppers, etc.)
* 1 cup cooked lentils
* ¾ cup garbanzo beans
* 10–12 sugar plum tomatoes
* ½–1 avocado, diced
* ½–¾ teaspoon turmeric
* ¾–1 teaspoon fresh-ground lemon pepper
* ½ tablespoon extra virgin olive oil
* 1–1½ tablespoons balsamic vinegar

1. In a large bowl with a sealable lid, combine the greens, cabbage, and veggies. Keep lentils, garbanzos, and tomatoes in separate jars. Add avocado and items in jars just before eating.

2. When you're ready to eat, combine 2 or more cups premade salad with 5 or 6 tomatoes and ½ avocado.

3. Sprinkle turmeric and fresh-ground lemon pepper, then toss with olive oil and vinegar.

HEALTHY HACK

For extra safety, look for balsamic vinegar that says "lead-free" on the label.

STEP 5 **Do Your Due Diligence on Dairy.**

Limiting animal products doesn't apply just to your favorite filets anymore. You gotta put dairy under the microscope, too. "I recommend limiting animal products, including cheese, yogurt, and milk, to 10 percent or less of your daily caloric intake," Dr. Fuhrman writes. "Ideally, if you do include animal products in your diet, limit the serving size to 2 ounces and not more than three times a week (up to 12 ounces total)."

So what's wrong with dairy staples? Studies have found that a diet high in moo products might have negative effects on health and up your risk of mortality.[26] There's also a *possible* cancer connection. Some research, including T. Colin Campbell's, has found evidence that casein, a protein in dairy, has carcinogenic effects in animal subjects and has been linked to some cancers in humans as well.[27] "Dairy is a very controversial subject," nutritionist Rachel Beller says. "High-fat dairy consumption has been linked to higher levels of estrogen and free estradiol in the body and a potential increased risk of breast cancer. However, it's not about

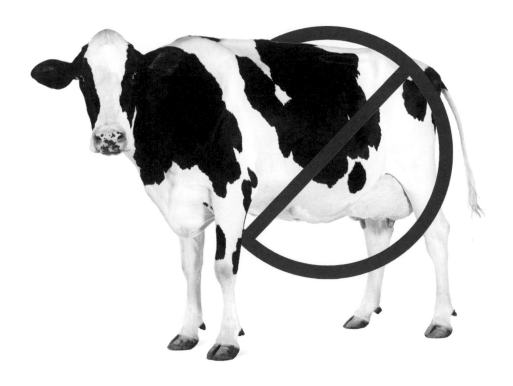

the fat itself but rather what's *in* the fat: hormones found in milk." In other words, the verdict on milk is murky.

All these dubious dairy effects compelled this cancer survivor to ditch the stuff almost completely. Again, you don't have to go vegan, but the science shows that it's better to limit your intake of animal products, rather than wolfing them down. If you do want to consume dairy or meat, Dr. Fuhrman suggests thinking of them more like a garnish than a main course.

When you've been raised on dairy, it can be hard to quit cold turkey. Try these small steps to make the switch totally painless.

* **Move away from the milk.** Mix your usual cow milk with a nondairy alternative. Start with a 2:1 ratio of dairy milk to nut or soy milk—unsweetened to avoid those sneaky sugars!—and gradually scale back until you're fully off the moo milk.
* **Banish butter.** This one broke my heart, but you can start slowly. When cooking, swap butter for extra-virgin olive oil or avocado oil. Both are healthy fats, but remember to use them in moderation. Water sautéing is also an option. When baking, sub the same amount of applesauce for the butter measurement.
* **Cut the cheese.** I'm a sucker for a good burrata, so this one was hard, too. Try to reach for dairy-free snack alternatives that are just as portable, such as an apple with peanut butter or a handful of protein-packed raw almonds with a clementine.
* **Limit your yogurt use.** A little is OK, if it's the right kind. Avoid the chemical, sugar-laden varieties in favor of plain organic low-fat Greek yogurt or organic low-fat kefir. Your gut will thank you for all those probiotics. Limit your intake to a couple of servings a week and alternate with chia seed pudding—chia seeds; nut, soy, or coconut milk; a little agave nectar, and Ceylon cinnamon, mixed together and placed in the fridge overnight—to start your morning on other days.
* **Sour on sour cream.** Use one of your weekly allowances of Greek yogurt as a sub for dishes where you'd usually add a dollop of this fatty condiment.

STEP 6 **Make Friends with Fat.**
As you saw, my old diet treated fat like the devil: no nuts, no avocado, no olive oil, no egg yolk. My aversion to it ran so deep that I actually lost a BFF over an argument about not using yolks in the chocolate chip cookies we were baking. Yeah, it was serious. (BTW, I have a great no-egg recipe if you want to eat only the raw dough. Just ask!)

The thing is, not all fats are created equal. Our bodies need fat in order to absorb certain vitamins and minerals, build cell membranes, clot blood, and move our muscles.[28] It's also a major energy source. Here's where you should stand on the different kinds.

Friendly Fats

Found in veggies, nuts, seeds, and fish, mono- and polyunsaturated fats (aka good fats) help raise good cholesterol and fight heart disease. A diet rich in friendly fats, including olive oil and fatty fish (such as wild salmon) in moderation, avocados, and flaxseeds, forms the basis for the expert-loved Mediterranean diet.

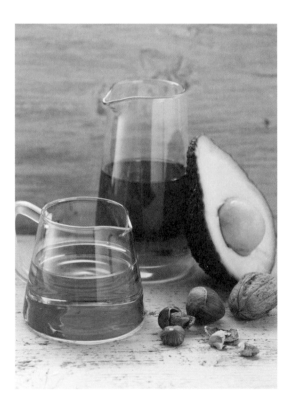

Frenemy Fats

Saturated fats are OK in your diet but only as acquaintances. You'll find them in foods such as red meat, dairy, coconut oil, and baked goods. Keep your consumption of sat fats to less than 10 percent of your total calories per day.[29] Remember, you're trying to limit your intake of animal protein anyhow.

Foe Fats

Trans fats are human-made monsters. They're found in processed foods linked to spikes in bad cholesterol and an increased risk of stroke, diabetes, and heart disease. Research from the Harvard School of Public Health found that for every 2 percent of calories from trans fats you consume daily, your risk of heart disease rises by a whopping 23 percent.[30]

STEP 7 **Open Your Eyes to Organic.** Any recipe ingredient you see in this chapter is part of your path to a healthier healthy, and selecting the organic versions of those ingredients, when you can, is the healthiest way to go. That means everything from fresh produce to packaged goods. I started with organic milk, then berries, and ran with it from there. Since committing to my healthiest healthy, I've made an effort to go almost totally organic for my produce.

Easier said than done, though, I realize. If you can afford to buy organic all the time

Dirty Dozen Always buy organic [31]	Clean 15 Usually safe to purchase even if not organic [32]
strawberries	sweet corn
spinach	avocados
nectarines	pineapples
apples	cabbage
peaches	onions
pears	sweet peas (frozen)
cherries	papayas
grapes	asparagus
celery	mangos
tomatoes	eggplant
sweet bell peppers	honeydew melon
potatoes	kiwi
	cantaloupe
	cauliflower
	grapefruit

for everything, go for it! If not, check out the chart on page 43 for the Environmental Working Group's list of the Dirty Dozen and Clean 15 (updated yearly). These lists indicate which products are the biggest offenders and which are relatively safe— organic sticker or not.

Keep in mind that a shiny "organic" badge on the package doesn't give you a free pass. Not all organic foods are healthy. Keep reading those nutrition labels and ingredient lists!

SHOP SAVVY

You've done a ton of research, gathered loads of expert information, and collected some ideas for a full plate makeover. Woohoo! But getting these items in your pantry becomes a whole different ballgame. The supermarket can be *super* overwhelming. Let's be real: Making some of these changes (*cough* buying organic *cough*) can also get pretty pricey. Here are some of my favorite frugal Frannie tips on how and where to shop smart and healthy.

* **Buy in bulk.** From parchment paper to bean-based pasta, bulk buys usually deliver the best value. If you can't store all those extra goods, split your order with friends or family.
* **Freeze your fruits and veggies.** Frozen organic fruit is a terrific and usually cheaper alternative to fresh.

* **Go generic.** These brands often offer the best bang for your buck, especially when it comes to pantry staples such as baking supplies or spices.
* **Clip coupons.** Take coupon clipping into the twenty-first century with #noshame by using apps such as Ibotta and Checkout 51.
* **Compare if you dare.** With a little legwork, you usually can find better pricing at less conventional grocery stores, such as Target or some of my other favorites listed below.
* **Stock up on savings cards.** If your grocery store offers a savings or membership card—and almost all of them do—get one. It's your free pass for discounts.

Where to Go

Confession: I get straight up *psyched* going to Costco. Showing the door guard my membership card and crossing the threshold into bulk heaven makes me want to break into song. Sometimes I'm tempted to use the shopping cart as my dance partner and glide up and down the aisles in full arabesque. (My kids are glad I don't.) The store employees join me at the chorus in three-part harmony. At the end, an explosion of confetti falls on me at the register . . . and *scene!* Yeah, I'm *that* much of a fangirl. It's a killer place for bulk discounts, and Costco offers a ton of organic options, from frozen fruit to pasta sauce—all at affordable prices. Here are some other online and in-store options where you can score a surprisingly wide array of healthy options and organic goods on the cheap(ish).

* Amazon
* Lucky Vitamin
* Sprouts Farmers Market
* Target
* Thrive Market
* Trader Joe's
* Vitacost

* Walmart (Yes, they sell organic)
* Whole Foods (Their 365 brand rocks!)

Shopping List

Stock up on these can't-live-without-'em pantry staples next time you hit the grocery store, and you'll take one small step closer to your healthiest healthy.

Take this book with you on your next trip to the grocery store. It's just like having a nutritionist in your basket or shopping cart, I swear.

❏ bean and rice chips	Beanfield's brand, my naughty-but-still-nice snack.
❏ bean-based pasta	Because life's too short not to eat pasta.
❏ chia and flaxseeds	Toss these in smoothies, salads, and baked goods for a fiber-filled antioxidant boost.
❏ extra-virgin olive oil	For just about every dang thing.
❏ green superfood powder	Garden of Life brand has organic.
❏ matcha green tea powder	The perfect superfood for sipping or smoothies.
❏ raw almonds and cashews	The perfect snack or salad topper.
❏ raw organic protein powder	Garden of Life brand—because where would my smoothies be without these?!
❏ wild tuna	Safe Catch Elite brand, a low-mercury lunch on the go, filled with omega-3s.
❏ sprouted grain bread	Food for Life Ezekiel 6:9 brand, a favorite for breakfast toast, as well as this brand's cereals and tortillas.
❏ unsweetened vanilla almond milk	Preferably without carrageenan.
❏ whole wheat pastry flour, coconut flour, and almond flour	Kick-ass ways to boost the health content of any baked goods.

THE SEVEN-STEP NUTRITION REVOLUTION

OK, I know we just went through a *lot* of info, so here's an easy-peasy, seven-step guide to revamping your refrigerator and purging your pantry.

STEP 1 **Skip the sucrose.**
Remember how sugar sneaks into everything from ketchup to salad dressing? Look at your labels and introduce those sneaky sugars to their fancy new home: Chez Garbáge.

STEP 2 **Forsake the fructose.**
Ditch anything that contains high fructose corn syrup. Read all the labels all the way to the end because this silent killer shows up in more than just the sweet stuff. Check your ketchup, cereals, pasta sauces, packaged goods, and drinks. It's a game of hide-and-seek, but you *will* win.

STEP 3 **Junk the juice.**
Juices are big diet deceptors. They seem healthy—and in some ways they are—but they also have tons of sugar and possibly added chemicals. Sip 100 percent juice, and for bonus points go for fresh-squeezed. Even when drinking fresh, limit yourself to no more than 6 to 8 ounces per day.

STEP 4 **Peter out processed.**
Packaged goodies with endless ingredients lists full of things you can't pronounce usually aren't going to do you any nutritional favors. Go fresh whenever you can.

STEP 5 **Can the cans.**
Aluminum cans can leach traces of metal or toxins into your food. Yikes! Swap your canned goods for boxed or glass-jarred ones when you, um, can.

STEP 6 **Toss the temptations.**
Yep, you see them, and that's exactly the point. Keep the junk food out of mind by keeping it out of sight in your pantry and fridge.

STEP 7 **Grab-and-go goodies.**
Make snacking easier on yourself—not to mention the kids—with precut fruit and veggies so they're ready when you're on the run or packing lunches. My fridge is a stage, and fresh fruit and veggies are the stars of the show. Every time we reach for a snack, those fresh, colorful jewels are standing front and center, ready to dance into our mouths.

RESULTS

Looking back, it's crazy to think how one small step—switching my morning yogurt to cut the sugar—led to such massive improvements in my body and mindset. That yogurt swap turned into a relationship

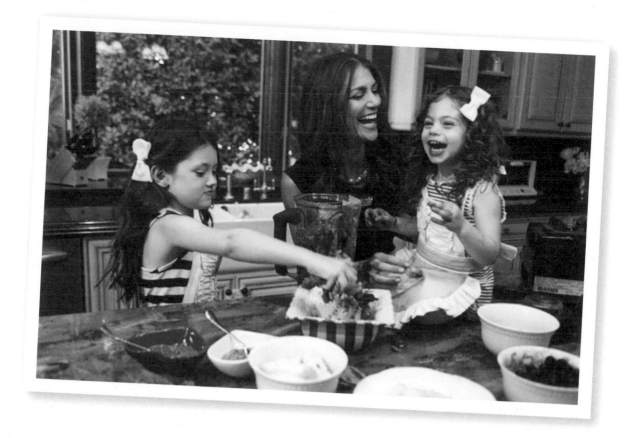

with chia seeds, which sparked a protein shakeup, an organic overhaul, and an animal-products purge. After a couple months of eating with plant-packed purpose, I noticed two tremendous transformations.

* **Weight loss.** Despite the *massive* portions of veggies and doses of healthy fats I was eating, I dropped some weight. I wasn't trying to, which was the best part, but as a by-product of these dietary alterations, the scale dipped down.
* **Incredible energy.** My verve totally swerved. I felt *great* with newfound, all-day oomph that has been truly life-changing!

For me, more energy equals more happiness. The kids don't get on my nerves as easily, and my patience radiates through the house. Even my skin looks brighter. This newfound exuberance totally surprised me. That's probably the biggest gulp of sweet, sweet lemonade that resulted from a bitter start in my search for a healthier me.

Now that I had my kitchen under control, I started to find ways to be healthier in a place I already thought I ruled: the gym.

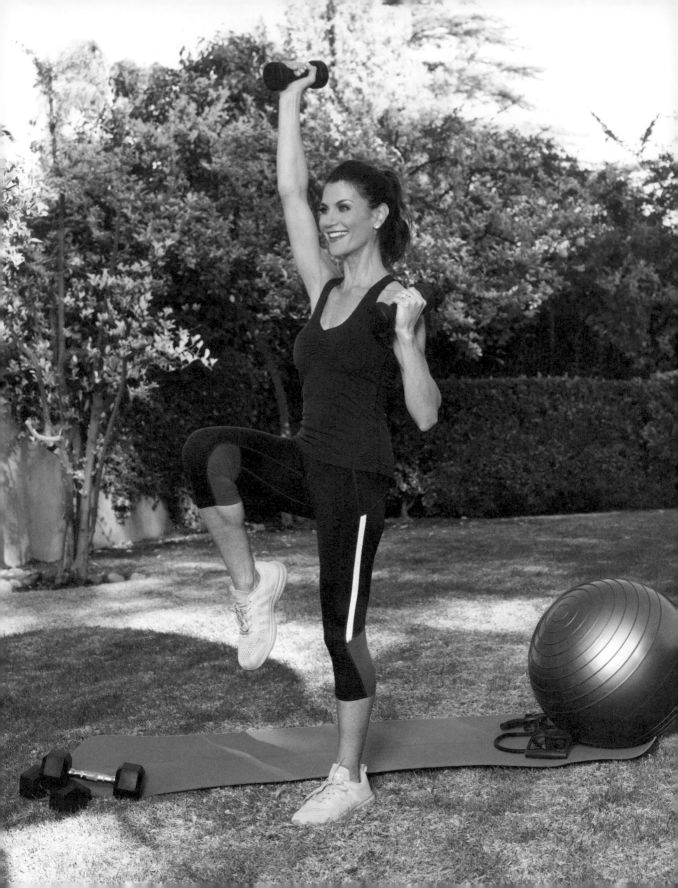

2

WISE UP YOUR WORKOUT

My fitness groove didn't hit its stride until my mid-20s. I've always been on the slimmer side, and, despite that childhood butter habit (*cringe*), my passion for dancing and a teen metabolism kept me in skinny jeans. But you wouldn't have called me a fitness freak then. I just did what I loved, high-kicking my heart out with the Hopkins High dance line and not worrying about body fat percentage or cardiovascular fitness.

In college, my inner nerd always kept me a week ahead on the required reading, and there was no daily dance team practice, so getting my butt in gear and into the gym proved difficult. Just like your biceps, motivation is a muscle. You have to build it, step by step. When I wasn't working my tail off in journalism school, Northwestern's dance program became my jam for twice-weekly, heart-pumping jazz classes, but my motivation was still dragging.

At 22, I weighed only a little more than I do now, but my love affair with deep-dish pizza left me dough-bellied and pudgy-faced. Never mind having the strength to handle the kinds of classes that I crush these days. This was my *un*healthiest healthy.

When I moved to L.A., my motivation finally started to kick into gear. It took some trial and error—skipping workouts to hang with friends, juggling three jobs while trying to catch my big break—but I took advantage of the city's great weather and robust fitness scene. A hefty dose of variety also kept my motivation flexin'. Once I started varying my workouts to keep my mind interested and my body guessing, I actually started to *like* working out. (I know, right?)

My romance with the gym started more as a comedy of errors than a hot and heavy love affair, though. I first joined the local ladies-only gym, ditching Jane Fonda for kickboxing and body sculpting workouts. I didn't know proper form for any of the basic exercise classes. In step class, I fell a handful of times, and, rookie move, I even locked my padlock key inside my gym locker. My groove slowly started to find its rhythm, but then a couple of years later a relationship derailed me. My sweat sesh often took a back seat to spending time with my new boyfriend. (Apparently, boys didn't have to be *in* my gym to affect me.)

The heartbreak of our breakup ironically put me back on track. In a desperate attempt to find some positivity in all that sadness, I realized that, by making my body feel happy and strong, my mind and soul began to feel confident and secure again, too. My relationship with my body was starting to become about how I felt rather than just how I looked. I still had a lot of learning to do, but I was approaching a healthier healthy.

As my broadcast career took off, talk shows started booking me as a fitness expert. Fitness magazines were putting me on their covers. Then, at age 32, I landed a dream gig cohosting *Dancing with the Stars*, the ABC prime-time hit. I kept working out hard—maybe even harder. Standing next to all those tanned, toned professional dancers was seriously intimidating, and it made me acutely aware of how my own body looked. Keeping up became a big priority and seriously boosted my motivation.

It paid off. Being around the pros prompted me to make my fitness hobby more of a professional pursuit. Magazines were interviewing me about my body,

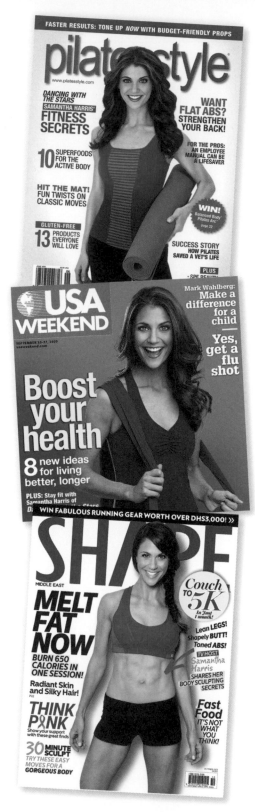

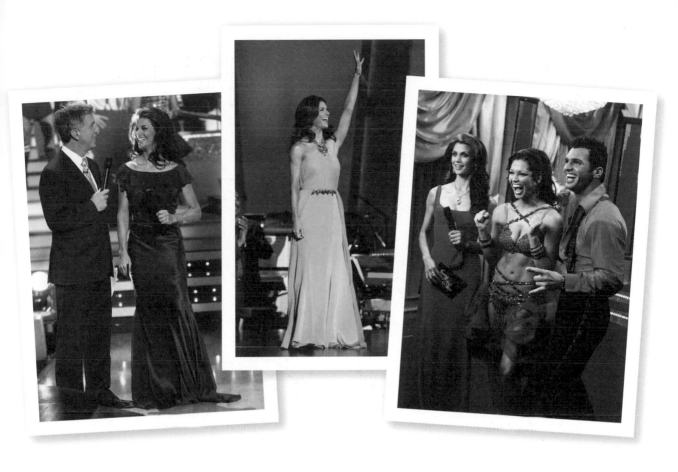

diet, and workouts, and my answers had to have as much credibility as possible. After an eight-season run with *DWTS*, and while on hiatus from *Entertainment Tonight*, I earned my credentials as a certified personal trainer. That's right, I'm Samantha Harris, CPT. Watch out, world! Seeing my hard-earned abs on the cover of *Shape* magazine (*so cool*) and being mistaken for a pro dancer were thrilling, I confess. That ego boost fueled my competitive streak even more—though maybe not for the healthiest reasons.

STAIRWAY TO BROADWAY

If *DWTS* was body boot camp, my next professional challenge was Navy SEAL combat training. A love of musical theater runs through my veins. My family and I did sing-alongs to *Fiddler on the Roof* and *West Side Story* when I was a kid, and I auditioned for every high school musical and musical variety show at my synagogue while growing up. I didn't pursue musical theater on Broadway, but then the stars aligned. Right before my last season on *DWTS*, a dream-come-true

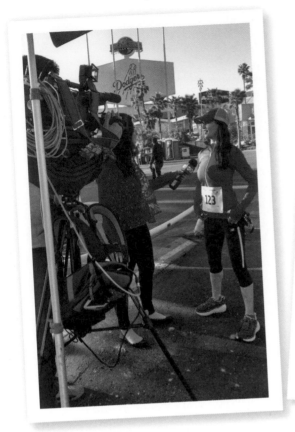

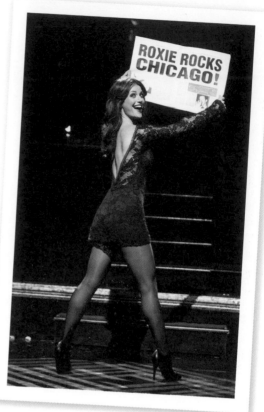

opportunity arose for me to do my best Fosse jazz-hands as Roxie Hart in *Chicago*.

I was in peak shape, but live theater—eight shows a week—requires a whole new level of stamina. Did I mention I was trying to balance *Chicago* with hosting duties at my other TV show, *The Insider*? Oh, yeah, and most of my fitness goals centered on *looking good*. Broadway is all about what you can do. Do you have the endurance and flexibility to make it through endless eight counts? Can you sing to the rafters while leaping across the stage? If I was going to make it through my opening night without collapsing, it was time to start measuring workouts by performance gains, rather than the mirror.

Good old-fashioned stair climbing got me ready for my Broadway debut. I strapped my 18-month-old baby to my back and went two-by-two up a flight of 40 stairs near our house, over and over and over, while belting out "Me and My Baby" from *Chicago* at the top of my lungs. The occasional horn honked as someone drove by, but I think people just assumed that moms do crazy things to get their babies to nap! Remember, in your healthiest healthy, it's not about the size of your thigh gap, it's what your body can *do*.

THE NEW NORMAL

You know all that research we've been talking about so far? How docs have shown that eating right and exercising right can help prevent cancer? After my diagnosis, one of my first thoughts was: EFF THAT. Nearly two decades of hauling my butt outta bed on Saturday mornings to get to the gym just to become an exception to scientific evidence and wind up in an oncologist's office? WTF?

After wallowing in pity and indulging in a therapeutic bonbon or two, I wised up. After many conversations with my doctors, it dawned on me that it was *because* I was so healthy that I found the cancer early. *Because* I was so healthy, I had a lower risk of complications in surgery. *Because* I was so healthy, I faced a faster recovery and reduced chances that this $#!% would come back.[1] Cancer wasn't going to sour my relationship with my body. I wasn't going to let it.

Lying in recovery for weeks on end made me appreciate my body and what it can do on a much deeper level. It was time to start paying attention to all the lovey-dovey mumbo-jumbo that my yoga teachers blathered about during class: Our bodies are crazy amazing. They literally carry us through life, so the least we can do is show them some love in return. We get only one body, so *slow down and listen to it*.

Turns out, this kind of inspiration—intrinsic motivation—will be your friend 'til the end. "Finding the deepest reason that you want to exercise is much more effective than doing it for external reasons—like looks," says Dr. Jonathan Fader, a leading sports psychologist and performance coach who works with NFL and MLB players. "An intrinsic motivator would be wanting to enjoy the time you spend with your grandchildren when you are older, or wanting to live longer for your family, or wanting to show your family what a healthy lifestyle is."

Check, check, and check.

FEEL-GOOD FITNESS

One location of my gym lies in an area known as Boys Town, so most of the guys there play for the other team. One day before a killer ass-burning class, all the buff hotties were standing outside, showing off their toned and tanned L.A. physiques. As I was ~~gawking~~ glancing at one particularly fit guy, he did something I still can't fathom. He pulled out a pack of cigarettes. We all know why lighting up has no place in your healthiest healthy, so don't make me belt out a "No Smoking" song for you. What really killed me, though, was that guy obviously cared about his body. He was in great shape and walking out of a *gym* for chrissake. But he clearly wanted a hot bod, rather than a healthy one.

Seeing that screwed-up health logic really riled me up. Remember, that's how I approached my own fitness for a long time. It was tough medicine watching that same impulse in action in someone else. Exercise has brought so many good things into my life, including ambition, confidence, and energy. The ambition to reach for the stars (sometimes literally), the confidence to pursue my dreams, and the energy to keep up with my dance-loving daughters. Finding my groove took time. First, I had to untangle all the old stereotypes about tight abs and thigh gaps to find a more meaningful, more effective motivation. It ain't always easy. But a beautiful part of finding your healthiest healthy is developing a better relationship with your body, your fitness, and yourself.

Do I still push myself in the high-intensity interval training (HIIT) classes? Hell, yeah! Much of what I do hasn't changed. But my attitude toward fitness has done a total 180. After cancer, looking toned is a nice side effect, but if my thighs get a little thicker because I'm kicking ass in kickboxing, then *bring it on.* In other words, you should hit the gym with mindfulness. Rather than doing yoga for sculpted arms, do it for the time to Zen out and take stock of how your body feels. What spots are sticky and need some lovin', and which muscles need a rest? Rather than pushing yourself to do 20 tuck jumps, hit 10 and then switch to something lower impact to preserve your joints. They need to last at least a few more decades! Rather than measuring your progress by numbers on the scale, look at indicators of overall health, such as body fat percentage, cholesterol levels, strength, and stamina.

Come on, you got this!

FITNESS FIRST

Rekindling your relationship with the gym—or just starting one—is about improving your health at its core, not getting six-pack abs. Here are 10 ways that exercise can improve your life from top to toe, along with how best to score each benefit.

1. Boost Your Brain.

Exercise can keep your mind sharp by improving your memory. A 2016 study published in *Current Biology* found that exercising within four hours of learning new info stimulated areas in the brain associated with memory, giving you a boost for recalling information.[2] Hitting the gym also can improve visual-spatial processing and attention skills.[3]

★ Aim for at least 75 minutes in the gym per week. (You'll need more time there, however, to improve other parts of your bod.[4]) Even a single sweat session can improve your ability to recall facts.[5]

2. Reduce Stress.

Work represents one of the biggest sources of stress in our daily lives. I effing *love* my career, but it still overwhelms me sometimes. Studies show that 60 to 90 minutes of exercise over the course of your day can help your body stop the stress cycle.[6]

★ Take a brisk walk on your lunch break. A 2015 study published in the *Scandinavian Journal of Medicine and Science in Sports* found that, if you take a 30-minute walk, you'll feel more enthusiastic about your work and better equipped to kill it in the afternoon.[7] Take that, boss lady!

3. Fight Depression.

After my first serious breakup, I turned to exercise for a good reason. Even light activity, such as going for a walk, has an antidepressant effect that can help you shake a funk.[8] To paraphrase *Legally Blonde*, exercise creates endorphins, and endorphins make you feel good. When you're having trouble getting your butt to the gym, think of it as happy hour for your brain.

★ Clear out those cobwebs. A 2016 study published in *Behavior Therapy* found that as few as 30 minutes of light, moderate, or intense physical activity significantly improved the mood of depressed women.[9] Hop on a stationary bike and watch a stand-up comedy special or an episode of your favorite sitcom. Better yet, get some fresh air and take a spin around the neighborhood.

4. Pump Your Heart.

Your heart is literally a muscle, and you gotta work it! According to a massive research review by the Sports and Exercise Council of the American College of Cardiology in 2016, the more you get your heart pumping, the more your risk for cardiovascular disease declines.[10]

✳ Even tiny tweaks can deliver a big heart-healthy boost, so switch to a standing desk, do walking lunges on your next conference call, or take the stairs instead of the elevator.

5. Up Your Energy.

You know that rush after a good workout where you feel like you could dance home? It seems counterintuitive, but gettin' your schvitz on gives you *more* energy, rather than less. Even crazier, you can achieve this energy boost in just five minutes—yeah, *five.* A 2016 study published in the *International Journal of Behavioral Nutrition and Physical Activity* found that taking a break every hour for a quick 5-minute walk made participants feel more energetic, happier, and less tired and hungry.[11]

✳ Twenty jumping jacks—right now!

6. Strengthen Your Bones.

A 2015 study published in the *Journal of Sports Medicine and Physical Fitness* found that low-weight, high-repetition exercise increased bone mineral density up to 8 percent.[12] That adds up as you start pitting

Mother Nature against Father Time—for postmenopausal women, that gain jumped to an amazing 29 percent!

✳ Grab the baby weights in spin class or challenge yourself to do more reps in the weight room.

7. Turn Back Time.

Scientists have found the fountain of youth—it's just past the locker room. In a 2015 study, researchers found that getting physical boosts your NRF1, a compound that protects your telomeres. In non-geekspeak, it slows the aging process.[13]

✳ Aerobic activity revs up blood flow, delivering oxygen and nutrients that improve skin health and help you keep your youthful glow. Work some jump squats into your next routine.

8. Sleep Better.

A killer exercise class can poop you out, but a regular, active routine can help improve your sleepy-time skills over the long haul. It's a chicken-and-egg situation, but a 2013 study conducted by researchers at Northwestern University found that participants slept better after four months of an established exercise routine.[14]

✳ Create a healthy routine and stick to it. No ifs, ands, or buts! Also prioritize good sleep because the effect seems to work both ways. Not getting enough sleep can make you more likely to skimp on or skip the gym the next day.

9. Sweeten Sex.

Exercise can seriously improve your sex life—just ask my hubby! But the benefits go beyond the confidence boost from feeling proud of your body. Just 20 minutes of vigorous exercise can increase a woman's physiological arousal.[15] Sexercise burns calories, too, but not enough to replace your workout. (Damnit!) A recent study found that women burn an average of about 70 calories over the course of a horizontal lambada.[16] That's the caloric equivalent of one banana. If you want to swap out your usual sweat session for something steamier, you'll have to get . . . creative.

✱ Pound out 20 minutes on the treadmill, hit the shower, and then it's *Fifty Shades of Grey* time!

10. Fight Cancer.

As a research-backed rule of thumb, more exercise = less risk of cancer.[17] That's partly because being overweight or obese increases the risk of certain cancers. One massive study of about 1 million Americans found that participants with higher BMIs were more likely to die than cancer patients with lower BMIs.[18] Physical activity can lower the risk of endometrial cancer by 20–30 percent, breast cancer by 25 percent, colon cancer by 24 percent, and ovarian cancer by 20 percent.[19] Exercise also aids in cancer recovery.[20] Researchers at Ohio State University did a study with more than 500 breast cancer survivors and found that those who stuck to an exercise regimen during and after treatment reported improved quality of life, less fatigue, and less pain.

✱ Talk to your doctors to see what kind of exercise(s) they recommend

FLEX YOUR MOTIVATION

To find your workout groove, try different workouts on different days and at different times. Record your energy level before, during, and after you sweat, says Delf Enriquez, CSCS and group fitness manager at Equinox Fitness Clubs. "Compare your results and try to schedule your workouts when you felt the best and had the most productive and effective workout," he says. "By doing this, you'll have better workouts, not get so tired afterward, and be more inclined to incorporate working out into your schedule."

Not every city has endless choices for workouts. But you can zone in on some Zen or catch a quick cardio session with the flick of a finger. A 2015 study found that people who used fitness apps boosted their leisure-time activity levels and had lower BMIs.[21] Plus, so many of the apps are free! (Cue celebratory shimmy.) Check these out to fuel your fire:

* **Aaptiv** offers an anywhere, anytime personal trainer that mixes a full-on guided workout with a get-in-gear playlist. Options range from 5 to 90 minutes, which will satisfy any workout need.

* **ACTIVEx** is perfect for group-class groupies because it plugs you into a community no matter where you're getting your sweat on. With Tabata-based (HIIT) exercises and training plans, this baby is a killer.

* **Amazon Echo's Alexa** might not be a drill sergeant, but she can still get you movin', double time. Ask her for a 7-minute workout, which will guide you through timed jumping jacks, wall sits, push-ups, squats, and other standard, great-for-you moves.

* **Down Dog** is a guided yoga session at the pace, level, and time frame you crave. It's my go-to whether I have 15 minutes or an hour.

* **MapMyRun** gives you no excuse to skip a workout when you skip town. Enter the zip code and the app will show you running routes in that area. It even has a Route Genius feature. Tell it how far you want to run and

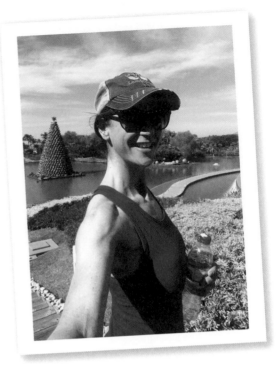

the app will generate a scenic route for you.

* **Seven** is the science-backed magic number with this app. Choose from a library of 7-minute workouts that use only a chair or wall and your body weight. No excuses not to get a hotel-room workout on your next business trip!

* **Sworkit,** short for "simply work it," lives up to its name. With videos for more than 200 types of exercise, all demonstrated by personal trainers, you can smash your goals by building strength, increasing flexibility, and committing to calorie-crushing cardio. They also have a special version just for kids.

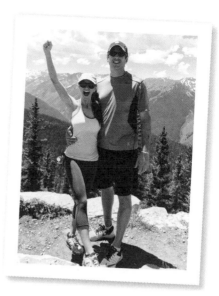

LIGHT THE FIRE AND KEEP IT BURNING

Deprioritizing the gym happens to the best of us, and that's not a bad thing! As Type A as I am about getting my gym time these days, I also don't beat myself up if I skip it to spend quality time with my sweet hubby—although I usually try to kill two birds with one stone by going for a run together with him. Creating a balanced schedule means building in flexibility. Just make sure you're not forgetting to take care of yourself, too.

STEP 1 **Schedule your workouts.**
Look at your schedule at the beginning of each week. Work, appointments, household tasks, kids, time for your partner, time for your friends, volunteering—oh yeah, and time for YOU. Put your workouts in black and white as weekly calendar appointments. Seeing that regularly scheduled sweat session pop up on your calendar makes it less likely that you'll find an excuse not to get your sweat on. Your workout, just like brushing your teeth, should form part of your normal routine.

If you don't have a full hour during the day to get to the gym, splitting it into two or three chunks still counts. A 20-minute yoga routine in the morning, a brisk walk at lunch, and a few rounds of burpees while you watch your favorite show at night. It's easier to manage than you think, and it all adds up! Try that for a week and see how you feel.

ANYWHERE, ANYTIME ROUTINES

When you're juggling a job, a relationship, a family and, you know, a *life*, getting to the gym can feel overwhelming. To make it easier, this chart from Heather King, CPT and the group training coordinator at Life Time fitness clubs, breaks down no-excuses-allowed

	5 Minutes	15 Minutes	
At Home	Jumping squats for 1 minute with a 20-second rest between sets OR Full-body stretch session	20 squats 10 push-ups 20-second plank 1 minute rest between each set	
At the Gym	As many reps as possible (AMRAPs) of your favorite exercise with lighter weights	Cardio intervals on the treadmill or stationary bike 2 minutes fast, 1 minute rest	
At the Office	Push your chair back and hold a squat for 60 seconds with 30-second rests between sets OR Jog up and down the stairs.	Kick your stairwell stepping up a notch and work in jump squats or star jumps.	
Outside	Walking lunges to your mailbox or the corner store and back	Add some squats and walking lunges while doing yard work or going for a walk in the park.	

workouts based on where you are and how much time you have. Remember, even just 5 minutes of cardio every day has body benefits![22]

30 Minutes	60 Minutes
10 wall slides 20 squats 20 high-knees 10 push-ups 10 lateral lunges on each leg 50 jumping jacks 30-second rest after each set and 1-minute rest after every 10 sets	Put your fave show on while alternating squats, wall sits, push-ups, and high-knees. Do planks and push-ups during the commercial breaks.
5 dumbbell squats 15 chest presses 15 single-leg toe touches 15 shoulder presses 15 dumbbell rows 15 lateral pull-downs 30-second plank 30-second rest after each set	Sign up for a group class and get movin'!
Take a walking lunch instead of a working lunch.	Try a fitness app in an empty conference room or turn your water-cooler gossip into a power walk with coworkers.
Saddle up and burn it out on your bike.	Hit the trails for a hike, go for a nice long run, or grab the family for a bike ride.

STEP 2 **Find Your Fitness Sweet Spot.**

What brings you the most satisfaction when you're sweating? Ask yourself a couple questions to find out:

* **What are your best workouts?** Think back to your last really awesome workout. Was it a killer new body-torching class you conquered, a race where you scored a new personal record, a yoga class where you didn't have to dip into child's pose for a breather, or a good long walk? Picture the feeling of total accomplishment that gave you.

_____

_____

_____

_____

_____

* **What makes those workouts memorable?** Now make a list of what makes your best workouts so good. Is it a shake-your-booty playlist? Being outdoors? Having tons of people around you keeping you motivated? Your own competitive streak? A drill sergeant instructor barking at you? The solitude to listen to your body?

_____

_____

_____

_____

_____

Research suggests that people who engage in personality-appropriate activities will stick with the activities longer, enjoy their workout more, and ultimately have a greater overall fitness experience," says Susan Davis-Ali, PhD, a social psychologist who developed a fitness interest profile test for Life Time fitness clubs.[23] Think about your answers to these questions as you take the quiz at the right to figure out if you're a workout introvert or extrovert.

Are you a fitness introvert or extrovert?

1. **Being in a workout class surrounded by people makes me feel:**

   A. **Self-conscious.** I'm sweating like a horse, and the instructor seems like a sadist.

   B. **Energized.** If the chick on the next bike is using the 3-pound weights, I'm *definitely* reaching for the 5-pounders.

2. **In yoga, savasana (corpse pose) makes me feel:**

   A. **Awesome.** I love the total stillness that lets me focus on my body after a challenging class.

   B. **Annoyed.** Couldn't we spend these 10 minutes swapping tips for nailing crow pose instead?

3. **Your BFF wants to go for a postwork run to chat. This sounds:**

   A. **Not ideal.** My runs are peak "me" time. As much as I love her, I hate the idea of having to ditch my headphones for chitchat. I'd rather catch up over coffee.

   B. **So fun.** The miles fly by when we shoot the breeze.

4. **A dance-based class should be:**

   A. **Quiet.** I like to focus on my movements in a calm, controlled environment, such as a ballet class.

   B. **Loud.** Club-ready beats and a peppy instructor make getting my groove on way more fun and engaging.

If you answered mostly or all A's, you're a workout introvert. Solo sessions are your jam.

If you answered all or mostly B's, you're a workout extrovert. Bring on the team sports and competitive classes. A study published in the *International Journal of Stress Management* revealed two awesome findings about group workouts: Working out with a crew boosted the calming, stress-reducing bennies you get from working out more than just sweating solo. It also made participants more tired because they likely were pushing themselves harder and tapping into that competitive fire[24]

If it's a mix of both, great for you. You have tons of options.

Best workouts for introverts

* **Solo runs** Sign up for a race, go it alone, and bring your headphones.

* **Power walks** A brisk walk is one of the best ways to get your heart rate up while clearing your head.

* **Solo gym sessions** Schedule your sweat sessions and make an awesome playlist so you can tune out during your squats and planks.

* **Yoga** The focus on, well, inner focus makes yoga the perfect class environment for a workout introvert to get in the zone.

Best workouts for extroverts

* **Group runs** Get the crew or some coworkers together to train for a 10k or plan group runs after work. I grab moms from school to hit the pavement after drop-off.

* **Gym buddy time** Enlist a pal to hit the gym with you a few times a week. You have someone to spot you, point out any weak spots in your form, and keep you accountable for showing up.

* **Cardio classes** There's nothing like learning a little choreography to feel like part of a team. If you're feeling ballsy, make a cardio dance class a date night alternative with your sweetie.

HEALTHY HACK

If the gym isn't your thing, don't worry. You can get going in lots of other awesome ways. A friend once roped me into a pole-dancing class, and it was super fun and made me move my body in new ways. If you know someone who does a great alternative workout routine, grab her and team up. If your kids are old enough, make it a family activity. (Well, not pole dancing!)

STEP 3 **Get into Your Groove.**
Another key part of any successful workout strategy is determining whether you thrive on a tried-and-true routine or crave shake-it-up variety. Take the following quiz to find out your style. (Singing Madonna's famous 1980s tune while you do it is strongly encouraged.)

Are you a routine queen or a variety vixen?

1. **What are your most successful workouts? When do you make it to every class, hit every goal, and feel like you can conquer the world?**

   _____

   _____

   _____

2. **Do you enjoy hitting the same place, machines, or classes over and over again? Do you prefer taking classes from the same instructor?**
   ❏ Yes ❏ No

3. **Do you like finding new running paths? Do you love using guest passes to try new gyms or maxing out your ClassPass options?**
   ❏ Yes ❏ No

If you answered yes to question 2 and no to question 3, you're a routine queen. Find a studio or apps you like and stick to them. When you're juggling a packed schedule, eliminating variables from the equation can make all the difference in achieving your goals. Skip the ClassPasses of the world and invest in a regular app or gym. Once you've found your favorite classes, make them standing appointments in your calendar so they become second nature.

If you answered no to question 2 and yes to question 3, you're a variety vixen—like me. Skip a traditional gym membership in lieu of something like ClassPass, which allows you to try a ton of different classes and studios each month. Download an app with a huge library of guided workouts so you can mix it up. If you do join a gym, look for one with a stacked roster of classes or, better yet, one that changes the class lineup every month. My club, Equinox, does both, which keeps me consistently fired up.

If you answered yes to questions 2 and 3, then keep on enjoying the best of both worlds. But if you answered no to questions 2 and 3, you've got some work to do! Spend a month trying each approach and see which one amps you up more.

The Spice of Life

Even if you're a routine queen, make sure you switch it up sometimes. Maintaining balance is key for a healthy body and longevity! Muscle memory is great for slipping back into crow pose after a yoga hiatus but not so great when you're trying to challenge your bod. Research shows that the more variety you have in your workout routine, the harder you'll work out and the more you'll ultimately enjoy it.[25] You'll also reduce overuse issues. If running is your thing, do that, but make sure you throw in a weekly yoga session to keep your body flexible and injury-free. If you like lifting, circuit training–style, make sure to schedule some cardio for equilibrium or speed up your circuits.

Here are my top tips to make any move a little more interesting and give your body a fun new challenge.

* Convert any exercise that uses both arms or legs into a single-limb move and challenge your balance.
* Switch up your circuit by busting your moves in a different order.
* Increase the weight and cut the reps OR decrease the weight and up the reps.
* Target the same muscle groups with different moves. For example, if you usually work your chest with push-ups, try a chest press instead.

* Balance on one leg while doing arm moves to engage your midsection and challenge you. A rockin' core is on its way!

STEP 4 **Listen to Your Body.**

The most important point to remember when it comes to creating a healthy and sustainable workout routine—*Are you paying attention?*—is tuning in to your bod. The harder you push, the more calories you burn, yeah, but you don't want to burn out. Trainers and bodybuilders love pushing to muscle failure, but overexertion can lead to trauma fast. "By training properly, you can *minimize* the chance of injury," says Noam Tamir, CSCS and founder of TS Fitness in New York City.

INJURY PREVENTION 101

Worrying about injuring yourself doesn't give you a free pass not to push yourself; you still need to kick your own butt, which is why listening to your body is a fine art.

* **Always warm up.** Give yourself a solid 5 minutes.
* **Start small and build up.** It's better to underdo it than to overdo it.
* **Pay attention to your form.** Bad form will put you on a fast track to injury. Check out a variety of YouTube trainer videos or ask your instructor to guide you. Also watch yourself in the mirror

when you're learning a new move or practicing moves you think you've got down. Make sure you've aligned yourself in all the right places.

* **Work with a professional.** If you have a preexisting condition or injury, you might be causing your body more damage, even if it feels OK while you're working out. A pro will make sure you work around those issues.

* **Foam-roll on the reg.** A good roll after your workout will help increase mobility.

When I got pregnant for the first time, I used a heart-rate monitor to make sure I could keep up with my regular workouts while keeping mommy and baby healthy and safe. Turns out the burn zone—the beats-per-minute ratio where someone of your age and weight torches the most fat— was way lower than I thought. Better yet, it was a pretty comfortable range of exertion. Before that, if my lungs didn't feel like they were about to burst, I thought I wasn't pushing myself hard enough.

To this day, that's one of the most valuable workout lessons I've ever learned: Always push yourself, but don't kick your own butt so hard that it turns black and blue. If this is exciting news, put down the book, stand up, and give me a booty-shake dance in celebration. See? Getting your heart rate up *is* fun!

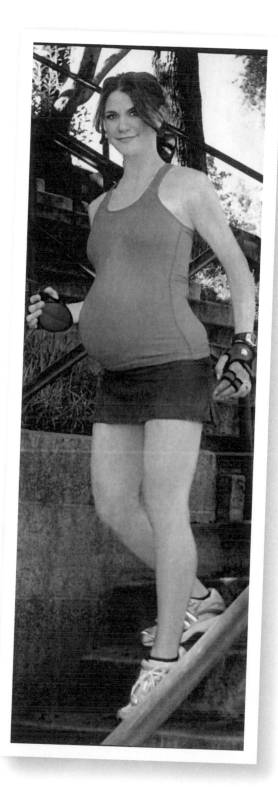

To figure out your personal healthiest heart-rate zones, use the equations below to calculate your maximum heart rate and then the subsequent pulse ranges.[26]

* In the fat-burning zone, you'll burn a greater percentage of calories from fat, though your overall calorie burn might be lower.
* The cardio zone is the best for peak heart health as well as great for calorie burn.
* Peak zone is best for short intense workouts, such as Tabata or other HIIT exercises.

HOW HARD IS TOO HARD?

Overdoing it can lead to short-term setbacks and long-term damage. Not your goal, my healthy friend. How hard is too hard? Let's take a look with Noam Tamir.

The Talk Test

If you can't talk comfortably during the majority of your workout, you're overdoing it. During an all-out Tabata session or sprint to the finish line, you're using your lungs to give it your all, but if you're too winded to speak once you pump the brakes, you need to dial it back.

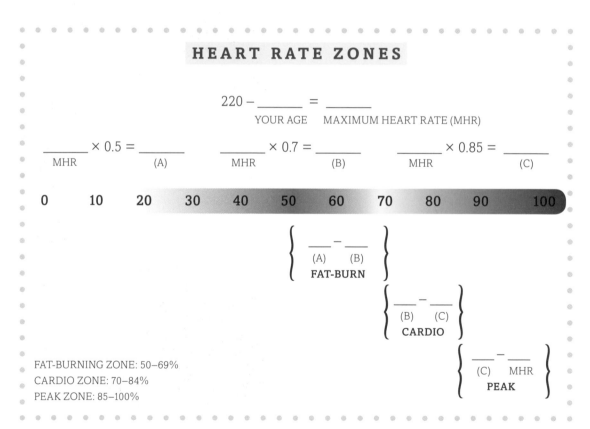

HEART RATE ZONES

$$220 - \underline{} = \underline{}$$
YOUR AGE   MAXIMUM HEART RATE (MHR)

$$\underline{} \times 0.5 = \underline{} \qquad \underline{} \times 0.7 = \underline{} \qquad \underline{} \times 0.85 = \underline{}$$
MHR   (A)   MHR   (B)   MHR   (C)

0   10   20   30   40   50   60   70   80   90   100

$$\left\{ \underline{} - \underline{} \right\}$$
(A)   (B)
FAT-BURN

$$\left\{ \underline{} - \underline{} \right\}$$
(B)   (C)
CARDIO

$$\left\{ \underline{} - \underline{} \right\}$$
(C)   MHR
PEAK

FAT-BURNING ZONE: 50–69%
CARDIO ZONE: 70–84%
PEAK ZONE: 85–100%

Measure Your Max

"Most people have an intrinsic sense of whether they can push harder," says Tamir. Picture your absolute max as a 10, like running a dead sprint to catch a connecting flight home for the holidays. Shoot for a 7 or 8 on that scale for a steady workout. Don't forget to adjust accordingly, either. If you're doing a quick 20-minute burn session, push a little harder. If you're working out for an hour, pace yourself.

Pay Attention to Pain

A knockout workout will make you sore, but serious pain might be telling you that you overdid it. "If you've been working out for a while and all of a sudden you have trouble walking or raising your arms the day after a workout, that's a good indication you overdid it," says Tamir. If the pain persists, see a medical professional who specializes in sports injuries.

WORKOUT LOG

Now that you know what you should be doing and how to do it, it all comes back to motivation. Reminding yourself of your workout highs can help you maintain your peak performance. According to the experts, recalling your positive physical activity–related memories encourages future workouts.[27] Keep notes on your calendar or right here. Consider this the first page of your OMG-I-Actually-Like-Working-Out Journal.

Exercise	Level/Speed	Time	Distance	Cals burned	Reps	Weight

Physical highs
Emotional highs
Goal for next time

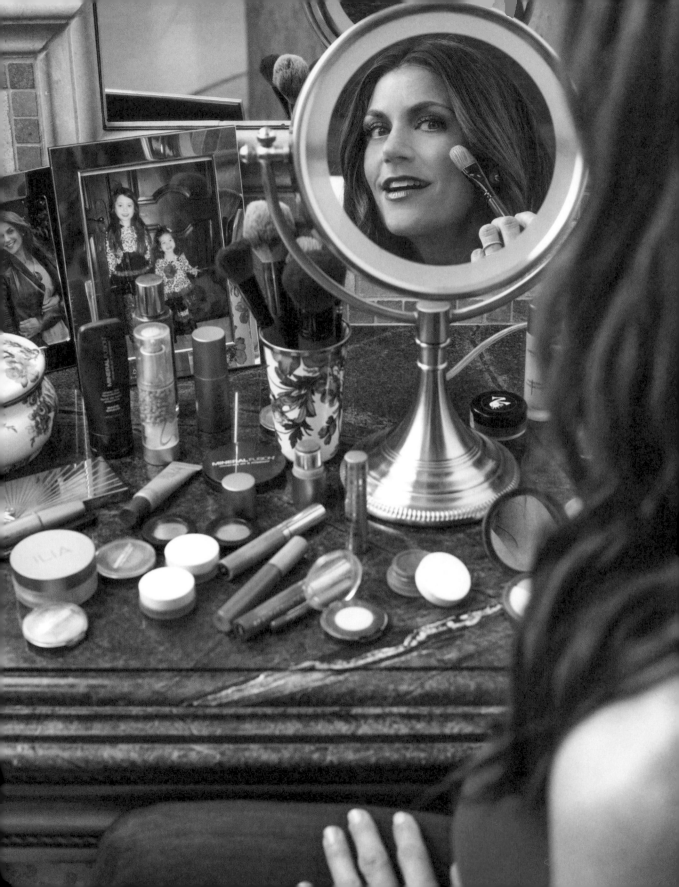

3

TAME YOUR
TOXINS

Now that my body and I were approaching the healthiest healthy phase of our relationship, I worried about what else it might be encountering. What's the good in treating your bod like a temple if you're plastering it with garbage?

I'm not one of those girly glowers who walks out of the gym with a dewy sheen. (What *is* their secret?) I schvitz . . . a lot. These days, I don't care about it, but, back in my mid-20s, a national tour of *Monty Python* songs and sketches (with Eric Idle!) required me to wear a skintight lavender bodysuit. Nowhere for sweat to hide. To keep that embarrassing, stain-making, pit pouring under control, prescription-strength antiperspirant lined my luggage. I slicked on so much aluminum chloride—the active ingredient in most antiperspirants—that my underarms became red and swollen. Pretty. But, heck, I was the only girl onstage without pit stains! Aluminum-based brands became my secret weapon for years.

Years later, with a TV career in full swing, my on-camera look required

bulletproof makeup and hair, and achieving that I-did-NOT-wake-up-like-this look included shellacking my face and spraying my hair solid. Fast-forward to my cancer diagnosis and my search for how it could have happened. Let me tell you, lemonade or no lemonade, I didn't want to part with any of the pretties in my beauty bag— even if they were serving up unhealthy

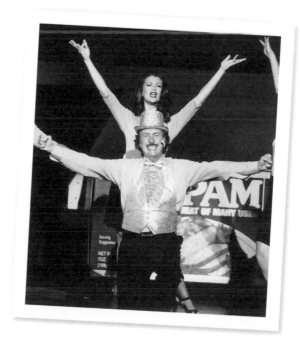

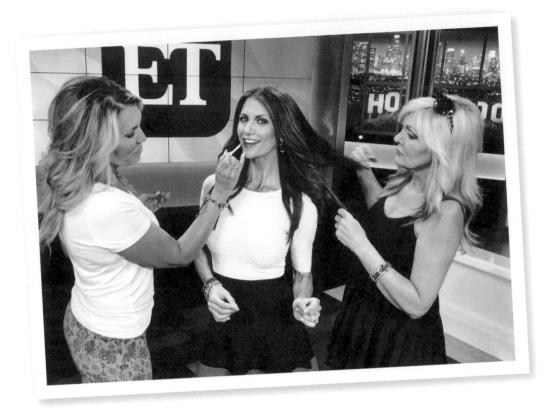

bitterness. Then something unexpected happened. So many breast cancer survivors asked if I had stopped using aluminum-based deodorants.

Um, nope. Why?

Turns out a lot of researchers think there could be a connection between your BO-stopper and breast cancer. According to the National Cancer Institute, there's no nail-in-the-coffin study saying the aluminum in your antiperspirant is *definitely* going to increase your risk of finding a lump, but studies have found that a disproportionately large number of breast cancers occur near the armpit, which has put scientists on alert.[1] The theory goes that aluminum on your underarms seeps through the skin and into breast tissue, where it potentially has estrogenlike effects—meaning cancer precursors.[2] The idea that my heavy-duty deodorant might have played even a small role in my encounter with the big C woke me up. How could something seemingly harmless enough to go on your skin daily be so potentially dangerous?

Back in the makeup chair at *Entertainment Tonight*, returning as a cancer survivor after a three-year hiatus, I started paying attention to my glammed-up TV look for more than just pro tips on applying shadow and keeping the contouring classy. The gorgeous glow from all those pricey highlighters and foundations sinking into my skin suddenly gave me a sinking feeling.

Turns out the average woman uses 168 chemicals on her skin every single day, so what other dangers were lurking in the medicine cabinet?[3] What about under the sink and in my home? I had detoxed my life from plate to push-ups, and then it dawned on me that what we put on and around our bodies matters just as much as what goes in them. It was time for a total toxin dump.

TOXIN DUMP 101

I'm not a chemist or an environmental scientist, so deferring to the scientists and experts made sense. After much Googling, I landed on a resource that's become my toxin-taming field guide and underlies many elements of this chapter: the Environmental Working Group, ewg.org.

They "empower people to live healthier lives in a healthier environment." Can I get a "Hell, yeah!"? (P.S. I totally wish I could steal that tagline as the subtitle of this book.) The EWG is a not-for-profit, nonpartisan group. Their work focuses exclusively on fielding questions with hugely impactful answers for your life, such as: "Is my deodorant going to give me cancer?"

Their publications aren't a bible for detoxing your life, but they come pretty damn close, which is why EWG's research and guides are the basis of so much of my personal journey and the advice here. The organization's stellar info, along with other guidelines in this chapter, will help you make the best choices possible on your journey to your healthiest healthy.

The EWG rates personal-care products on a scale of 1 to 10, 1 being the cleanest and 10 the most toxic. It's hard to shake that being a "perfect 10" is *not* desirable here, but that's the numerical rating system we'll use in this chapter. They give home products letter grades, "A" through "F," as in high school. (I got mostly A's then, so why change that now?—*cough* brown-noser, I know.) Even as my toxin-tapering Torah, the EWG isn't omniscient. They can't rate every single product on the market. Plus, the score they assign to a product averages each individually rated ingredient. So use the charts in this chapter thoughtfully to double-check ingredients lists and make informed choices, my healthy friend.

PURGE THE PARABENS

When it comes to your skin, the top toxic target is fairly well known: parabens. Walk down any beauty aisle, and you'll see bottles and tubes proudly labeled "paraben-free." That said, a ton of products you use daily still contains them.

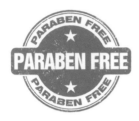

Parabens are endocrine disruptors, a class of chemicals that interferes with the hormone systems in your body. They chemically mimic estrogen and throw things out of whack to the tune of cancer, birth defects, and developmental disorders.[4] Yeah, not good. According to the Campaign for Safe Cosmetics— which works with breast cancer research partners and is also a great resource— products with a high water content, such as shampoo and facial cleanser, commonly contain parabens.[5]

A 2015 study conducted by researchers at the University of California at Berkeley found that parabens might increase your breast cancer risk more than scientists originally thought. Most studies have tested the effects of parabens on cancer cells solo, but in real life other factors come into play, such as growth hormones that occur naturally in your body. After testing the effects of parabens on breast cancer cells with different types of hormone receptors, researchers found that, when combined with a growth factor naturally found in your breast cells, it took just a measly 1 percent of the parabens to stimulate breast cancer growth. In laymen's terms: Parabens are *more* carcinogenic in real life than they are in the lab.[6]

Applying any product with parabens— lotion, sunscreen, foundation—can cause UV-induced damage to skin cells and screw with their growth rate.[7] No bueno. Certain parabens also have been linked to reproductive issues in animal studies. One such study found that exposure to butylparaben while pregnant or breastfeeding could alter the development of reproductive organs in the child.[8] Ack!

Given all these nasty side effects, it will shock you how many products still contain parabens—everything from your eye cream to your conditioner. Toss them all.

HEALTHY HACK

For some of the higher-end items that you can't bear to trash, vow to finish them and then make that the *last* time you buy them. Small steps!

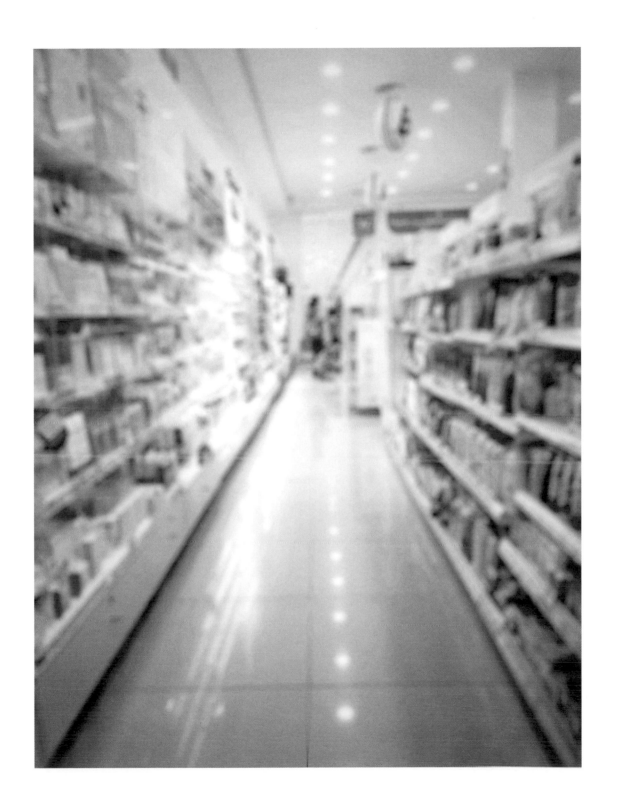

THE KEEP-OFF-YOUR-BOD LIST

Ingredient	What It Is	Why It's Harmful
*Parabens, most common forms: methylparaben and propylparaben	Chemical compounds used as a preservative in everything from shampoos to lotions.	Linked to breast cancer, skin cancer, and reproductive issues.
*Phthalates[9]	Usually hidden under the catch-all term "fragrance" on ingredient labels, they're in everything from conditioner to cosmetics. Toxins more often give the desired alluring smell of many products rather than, say, tuberose petals.	Linked to reproductive issues and early puberty. Experts worry that their endocrine-disrupting effects might play a role in breast cancer. Fragrances also can cause allergies and dermatitis.
Aluminum[10]	The active ingredient in many sweat-stoppers.	It's a bioaccumulative neurotoxin that collects in fat cells and destroys nerve tissues; also linked to Alzheimer's.
*Triclosan[11]	Antibacterial ingredient found in hand sanitizers and liquid soaps. Classified by the government as a pesticide.	Endocrine disruptor specifically shown to interfere with the thyroid. Also helps cause bacterial resistance to broad-spectrum antibiotics.
Formaldehyde[12]—may also appear as DMDM hydantoin, imidazolidinyl urea, diazolidinyl urea, quaternium-15, bronopol, 5-bromo-5-nitro-1,3-dioxane, or hydroxymethylglycinate	Smelly stuff from anatomy class found in foundation, soap, nail polish, hair-straightening treatments, and other products.	Classified by the International Agency for Research on Cancer and other agencies as a known human carcinogen.
1,4-dioxane[13]	A by-product of the process that makes certain skincare ingredients, such as petroleum, less irritating. This carcinogen is found in almost half of all cosmetics.	Linked to cancer and respiratory issues.
Polyethylene glycol (PEG)[14]	Often found in cleansers, conditioners, sunscreen, and moisturizers.	PEGs themselves aren't that bad, though they have been shown to cause irritation. The worry is that they're easily contaminated with ethylene oxide, a known carcinogen, and 1,4-dioxane, a possible carcinogen.

Ingredient	What It Is	Why It's Harmful
Products ending in –eth,[15] **such as ceteareth and triceteareth**	Typically found in anything that hydrates, including moisturizers or conditioners.	Similar to PEGs, these have a high risk of contamination by scarier ingredients.
Petroleum (mineral oil)[16]	Often found in moisturizers, petroleum jelly, and mineral oils.	Nontoxic when properly refined, they can be contaminated with PHAs, which are linked to breast cancer.
***Oxybenzone and octinoxate**[17]	Active ingredient in synthetic chemical sunscreens.	Associated with photoallergic reactions, cardiovascular disease, and potential cell mutations.
Ethanolamines[18] **MEA, DEA, TEA)**	Used as pH balancers, this group of chemicals is found in hair dye, mascara, foundation, fragrances, sunscreens, and more.	These chemicals can collect on and in your body and are linked to cancer, allergies, and potential birth defects.
Coal tar[19]	A derivative of coal, this is used in synthetic dyes and as an antidandruff agent in hair care products.	Like coal, a known carcinogen— especially through skin exposure.
Talc[20]	A mineral substance in everything from baby powder to shimmery eye shadow.	Linked to endometrial and ovarian cancer; also can be dangerous if inhaled.
Isobutane[21]	A propellant used in aerosol sprays.	A known carcinogen linked to reproductive issues; especially troublesome when inhaled.
***Phenoxyethanol**[22]	A preservative often used as an alternative to parabens. Sometimes also found in fragrances.	Classified by the European Union as an irritant and as potentially toxic in products used around the mouth.
Retinyl palmitate[23]	A vitamin A derivative found in anti-aging products and acne fighters.	Linked to skin cancer and possible reproductive issues when those using it are exposed to the sun.

*An endocrine disruptor.

I know, I know—these chemicals are bad, but purging them all and finding healthy replacements are way too much work, right? Plus, you don't want to break up with your favorite brands. Raise your hand if you're tempted to blow off all this info. Not too long ago, my hand definitely would have gone up, too. Even as a health and wellness nut, I spent years brushing this stuff off as fringe science or hippie BS. The ills of skincare nasties have been known and publicized for a while, but when you use a product every day and everything still looks fine, it's *way* freakin' easier to ignore the info than to part with your beloved beauty balms.

I get it. I really do.

But get this. Scientists and other experts have *proven* the sometimes carcinogenic consequences of these products. Your eye shadow looks nice, yeah, but do you want it to help turn you into a statistic? If you haven't been through the cancer shitshow, thank goodness for you, and let's keep it that way, my healthy friend! As hard as it is, taking these small steps is totally worth it. Do it one product at a time.

REQUIRE REGULATION

The more research I did on the overwhelming world of toxins, endocrine disruptors, and hormone inhibitors, the more it became clear that regulatory agencies don't have the power or money to keep these toxins out of the products we trust—and big corporations have too much money-hungry power. The federal Food, Drug, and Cosmetic Act, the final word on consumer-product regulations in America, hasn't been updated substantially since 1938. Seriously!

To give you an idea of how screwed up that is, right now the FDA bans or restricts only 11 chemicals in products sold in the USA. Compare that to the European Union, which has banned more than 1,300 chemicals and restricted almost 300 more.[24] In 2015, Senators Dianne Feinstein (D-California) and Susan Collins (R-Maine) cosponsored a bill called the Personal Care Products Safety Act, designed to make some much-needed twenty-first-century updates to regulatory standards. The bill would:

* Require the FDA to develop and implement cosmetic manufacturing standards consistent with existing national and international standards.
* Require cosmetics companies to allow the FDA to inspect their cosmetic safety records.
* Require the FDA to recall cosmetics likely to cause serious adverse health consequences, such as cancer or birth defects.
* Encourage the cosmetics industry

to use safety testing practices that minimize contamination.

But the bill is still stuck in Congress, which unfortunately means that you can't trust regulatory agencies to have your back here, so be your own advocate and step up to the plate when it comes to protecting your bod!

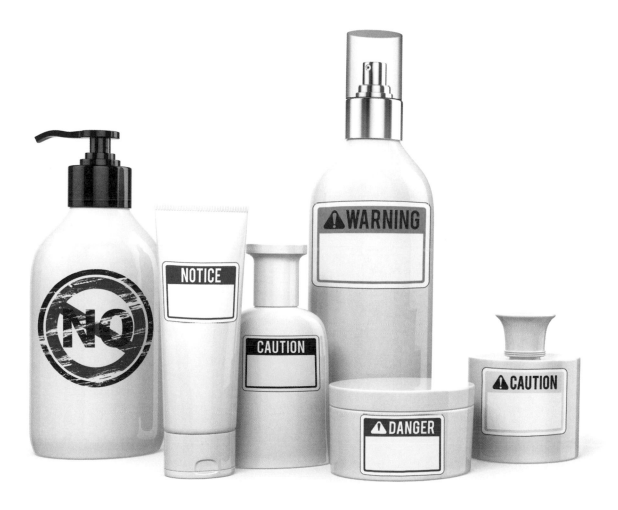

MOTHER NATURE'S SKIN SAVERS

More top derms and skin whisperers are turning to good old-fashioned beauty balms that you probably already have in your kitchen. Sometimes, you really can't beat Mother Nature for shiny hair and glowing skin.[25]

Ingredient	Where to Use It	Beauty Benefits
Honey	Honey-boosted facial masks are perfect for hyping up your skin.	This syrupy salve is one of nature's best sources of skin-boosting enzymes, vitamins, and balancing acids. Its antimicrobial properties help zap breakouts and balance moisture, and it even helps reduce scars.
Apple cider vinegar	If you can stand the stink, use as a facial toner or mix with water and sip as a morning tonic for a metabolism-boosting lit-from-within glow.	Vinegar's antibacterial, antifungal, and antiviral properties help banish blemishes; when imbibed, it helps balance bacteria in your gut and works wonders in countering heartburn.
Coconut oil	Use this sweet-smelling salve as a makeup remover (my nightly go-to), highlighter, shine-booster, even a full-body moisturizer. Also awesome for cuticle care.	Coconut oil is rich in natural antibacterial, antifungal, and antioxidant properties, which makes it awesome for strengthening skin and removing dead skin cells.
Tea tree oil	Awesome anywhere you have acne or redness.	This ancient Australian oil is a proven acne and inflammation fighter, thanks to its antimicrobial and antibacterial chops.

Ingredient	Where to Use It	Beauty Benefits
Sea salt	The stuff that scrub dreams are made of. Great for masks and toners, too.	Sea salt is a natural, mineral-rich, full-body exfoliant useful for sloughing off dead skin and stubborn rough patches. It also contains anti-inflammatory properties to soothe skin, reduce irritation, and help even out oil production.
Extra-virgin olive oil	The goodness of this pantry staple extends way beyond the kitchen. Use as a conditioning mask for your hair or a natural eye-makeup remover.	Hello, mega moisturizer! In addition to making skin smooth and strands shiny, some in the medical community believe it can help make hair thicker and stronger.[26]
Avocado	Use this green goddess as a moisturizing hair mask or skin softener and soother. But make sure you're not allergic first, as my poor BFF found out in seventh grade during our homemade face-mask experiment!	The good fats in avos are just as good for your skin as they are for the rest of your body; vitamins A, D, and E help soothe sunburn and boost collagen production.

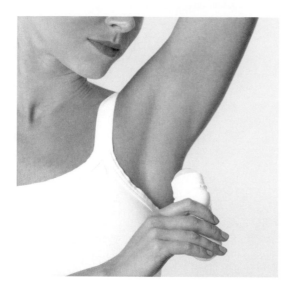

MAKEUP MAKEOVER

Brace yourself because this part can feel discouraging: The EWG list ranks many of the big brands in drugstore beauty aisles or at fancy-schmancy department store counters high—meaning super toxic. Ditto on the Think Dirty app, another awesome resource you should use for finding clean cosmetics.

So many women have to slap on a face at dawn that will last through high-pressure meetings, power lunches, playdates, happy hours, and PTA pow-wows. We need stay-all-day beauty that passes muster with hard-core eco-friendly beauty bloggers. Here's how to get your glam on without the toxic intake. These brands, available online or at select specialty beauty stores, are free of nasty skin saboteurs and will keep you glowing, on-camera or off. (Check out the Resources section on page 201.)

* Acure Organics
* Annmarie Gianni Skin Care
* Beautycounter
* Gressa
* Hush + Dotti
* Hynt Beauty
* Ilia Beauty
* Jane Iredale
* Jillian Dempsey
* Juice Beauty (also GOOP by Juice Beauty)

DEODORANT DISCOVERY

Your relationship with whatever you're putting on your pits probably isn't as deep and meaningful as your relationship with all the goodies in your glam bag, so this is an easy place to start taming those toxins. After learning about the ills of aluminum, that's exactly what I did, making a beeline for the natural beauty section at my local Whole Foods to find better options.

Not all green brands work, and the stinky, stained clothes from my own testing prove it. After some trial and error, here are my four favorites, none of which left me smelling like a hulking man:

* Crystal Essence (my fave)
* Fatco Stank Stop Deodorant
* Primal Pit Paste
* Simply Fair Coconut Oil Deodorant Balm

* Kjaer Weis
* Mineral Fusion
* Mineral Hygienics
* No Miss Cosmetics
* RMS Beauty
* TruFora Skincare
* Vapour Organic Beauty
* W3LL People

HEALTHY HACK

Some great mineral-based bronzers, blushes, and eye shadows don't look so hot on camera, so here's a little cheat. If you need a higher impact look or can't part with a "dirtier" brand yet, create a base with the clean product(s) before layering on the more questionable stuff. Think of it as a makeshift barrier between your skin and the toxins.

HAIR CARE OVERHAUL

Hair stuff is saturated with more toxins than McDonald's is with saturated fats. Products that promise ad-worthy hair often fall on the naughty list, but you don't have to get your hair in knots over this, promise. Here are two small steps you can take to tame the toxins in what you put on your tresses.

* Remember those nasty isobutanes from the chart on page 77? No good. Look for nonaerosols whenever you can. Try loose-powder dry shampoos in lieu of the propelled junk, natural Argan or Moroccan oil instead of a shine spray, and good old-fashioned squirt-pump hairsprays.
* Return to the chemical chart on page 76 to level up and start reading the ingredients lists on your more complicated products.

From shampoos to stylers, these clean brands have good locks on lock:
* Acure Organics
* Alaffia
* Attitude
* Avalon Organics
* Beauty Counter
* Carina Organics
* Free & Clear
* Honest Company
* Intelligent Nutrients
* Jason
* John Masters Organics
* Rahua
* Yarok

NAIL YOUR NAILS

One whiff will tell you that nail polish often contains lots of chemicals, and you may have heard of "5-Free" nails,[27] which refers to five nasty chemicals that you shouldn't be painting on your pointers.

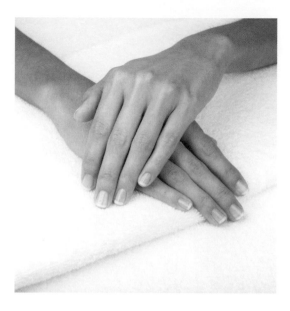

* Smith & Cult*
* RGB (vegan, cruelty-free, gluten-free, fair-trade)
* Zoya* (vegan)

*Also free of TPHP, a possible hormone disruptor, and Xylene, which is toxic when inhaled.[29]

SUNSCREEN

Because they have to stick to your skin while you sweat, as well as block the sun's intense UV rays, sunscreens often contain heavy-duty stuff that soaks through your skin and gets into your bloodstream.[30] The nasty stuff includes chemicals, such as oxybenzone, avobenzone, octisalate, octocrylene, homosalate, and octinoxate—all endocrine disruptors—and retinyl palmitate, a form of vitamin A that's potentially harmful to skin when . . . *wait for it* . . . exposed to the sun.[31] Kind of defeats the purpose, no?

In sunny Southern California, my family and I spend a lot of time outdoors: walking to school, playing in the park or the pool, driving with the sunroof open. We slather on a *lot* of sunscreen, so cheap is right on the money, honey. One of our friends always sends her kids to our house for summertime fun with their own sunscreen perfectly sealed in a plastic storage bag (#SuperMommy alert). She's so fancy. Me? I used to use the big-ass generic bottle of whatever was cheapest at the corner drugstore.

The nefarious five are toluene, linked to birth defects and nervous system issues; DBP, linked to cancer and reproductive issues; formaldehyde, a known carcinogen; formaldehyde resin, a by-product of the stronger stuff that still can cause irritation; and camphor, also linked to irritation.[28] Keep your claws chemical-free with these no-guilt nail brands.

* Deborah Lippman*
* Ella + Mila* (cruelty-free, vegan, fair-trade)
* Julep
* Kure Bazaar (cruelty-free, only 15 percent synthetic ingredients)
* LaCC (cruelty-free, vegan, gluten-free, paraben-free)
* Pacifica*
* Priti NYC*

Once my diagnosis made it clear that this stuff was important—like, *life-and-death* important—I hopped on the EWG's website to see how the big-brand and generic sunscreens stacked up. Ghastly. Even some baby-focused sunscreens, which you'd think would be safe and gentle because *duh*, had ratings of 10. Yikes!

I'm not here to shame you into prepping your own kid-friendly sunscreen bag or throw you and your sun-care routine some disapproving side-eye. Way too much mom-on-mom shaming happens already, so none of that here. My SuperMommy friend never did that to me, but I do wish she'd told me why she went to all that trouble to make sure her family was getting green 'screen. Because ultimately it's about making the right choices for YOU. Take what works for you and come back for more baby steps.

Thankfully, you can choose from a lot of sunscreens rated as 1s and 2s by the EWG. Most of them are mineral-based, which allows Mother Nature to take over for the mad scientists. The downside? They sometimes leave you looking like Casper the Friendly Ghost—a bit of an adjustment for any bronzed sun worshippers out there. In my healthiest healthy, I choose safety over looks every time . . . and this girl grew up using tinfoil reflectors and SPF 4 to tan. So get ready for your healthiest, alabaster beach bod! Kidding . . . sort of. Look for

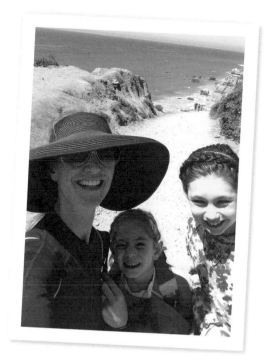

these sunscreens (available at major drug stores and chains such as Target or online) the next time you or your little ones are going to soak up some sun.

* Acure Organics
* Alba Botanica Mineral Sunscreen
* ATTITUDE Family
* Babo Botanicals
* Babyganics
* Badger
* Bare Republic
* California Baby Super Sensitive Tinted SPF 30
* The Honest Co. sunscreen stick
* Kabana Green Screen
* ThinkBaby (Especially Everyday Face—it's tinted!)

Remember that aerosol spray contains isobutanes, so if any of the recommended brands offer that option, don't buy it. Some have pressurized or pump sprays, a safer choice, yes, but they still pose an inhalation hazard—yuck. Creams and sticks are *always* the safest choices.

HEALTHY HACK

If looking pasty terrifies you, add some safe-choice tinted BB cream to a good SPF—or find some fashionable SPF 50+ rash guards. Ooh la la, so chic!

HEALTHY HACK

Don't forget your lids! In one UK study, researchers found that 77 percent of people miss the eye area when applying sunscreen—and, yes, you can get skin cancer there, too! If you're wary of slathering SPF on your eyes, try a mineral eye shadow or rock some good Jackie-O sunglasses all day.

PERIOD PURGE

Now that we've tamed the toxins going onto your body, let's look at what you're putting *in* your body. Join me as we, ahem, dig all up in the world of period poisons.

For starters, tampons *definitely* can be toxic, thanks to a gross cocktail of pesticides and bleach. Blech. Most big-brand tampons that include cotton also include the pesticides used to grow the super-absorbent white stuff, which winds up in the final product.[32] On top of that, they also bleach tampons made of cotton or synthetic fibers, such as rayon or nylon, to achieve that pure white we like. As a by-product, that chemical process produces dioxin, a toxin used in the Vietnam War weapon Agent Orange.[33] (I'm sorry, WHAT?) Dioxins are a known endocrine disruptor, shown to cause immune system issues and—you guessed it—cancer.[34] That's some serious shit going into your lady parts! Thanks to crappy legislation, tampon manufacturers don't have to dish on what they put in their products. It could be cotton or more likely rayon (a synthetic fiber made from sawdust, *ick*), viscose, or wood-fluff pulp mixed with chemicals.[35]

If you do only one thing from this chapter, trashing toxic tampons will have a mighty impact. Your skin is not only the largest organ in your body—as my then–six-year-old reminded me (hooray, kindergarten!)—it's also super permeable, especially the super-sensitive skin on your

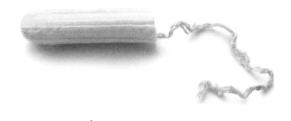

flower.[36] Anything in constant contact with it will make it into your bloodstream. The average woman uses 20 tampons per cycle, so that's like sticking at least 9,000 chemical suppositories up your vaj in a lifetime![37]

Even if you're not inserting something into your hoo-ha, the pads cozying up to your cooch can prove problematic, too. In 2014, Women's Voices for the Earth, a consumer advocacy group, tested a bunch of pads from the Always brand and found that the sanitary napkins emitted chemicals such as styrene, a carcinogen as classified by the World Health Organization; chloroform, a carcinogen, neurotoxin, and reproductive meddler; and chloroethane, a chemical known to cause lack of muscle coordination at high exposure, according to the FDA.[38] All of those are staying far away from my vajayjay, thankyouverymuch.

But what's a girl to do, short of free-bleeding?—and props to you women who do! I'm all about natural these days, but even that's a touch too far for me. Here are four small steps you can take to polish up your period routine.

* Swap out your toxic tampons for 100 percent organic cotton.

* Try 100 percent organic cotton pads at night when a little extra bulk won't bother you as much, or use thinner 100 percent organic cotton liners (from brands such as Rael) for daytime.

* If you're worried about the stay-put power of a natural brand, pop an organic pad into some period panties. Yes, Virginia, they're real: They have a pocket that holds the pad in place so you can strut onward with confidence.

Secret Toxic Chemicals in Pads

EXPOSURE CONCERNS:
reproductive harm
cancer
allergic rash
hormone disruption

pesticide residue ————————

dioxins and furans ————————
from chlorine bleaching process

adhesive chemicals ————————

fragrance chemicals ————————

* Go fragrance-free. Fragrances make feminine care products—wipes, sprays, tampons, pads—worse. Research from George Washington University found that fragrances in your lady business increase your exposure to endocrine-disrupting phthalates.[39]

HEALTHY HACK

Noncotton tampons are super absorbent but also tend to shed little bits of fiber into your vaj, upping your risk for toxic shock syndrome.[40] Organic cotton tampons, on the other hand, consist of tightly woven cotton that doesn't shed. They aren't quite as absorbent, so the ride might be a little shorter with these guys, but they're much safer and do the job just fine.

Even though the natural brands sometimes can feel like you traded a Porsche for a Prius, your chemical-free conscience and cooter will thank you! Plus, Priuses are cool now, no? Look for these tampon brands.
* BON
* The Honest Co.
* LOLA
* NatraCare
* Rael
* Seventh Generation Free & Clear

* Tampon Tribe
* TOTM

If you freak at the idea of sticking anything foreign into your bits, these reusable pad brands, available online at their own websites as well as on Amazon, deliver safe, cost-saving benefits.
* Charlie Banana
* Domino Pads
* GladRags
* Luna Pads
* Party in My Pants
* Sckoon Organic

For my free-bleeding friends or anyone who wants some extra backup on heavy days, these manufacturers make period panties (available online) that you may want to add to your arsenal.
* Anigan
* Dear Kate
* Knixwear
* Lunapanties
* ModiBodi
* THINX

The Queen of Cups

With these cleaner choices under my belt (wink), it was time for the big guns: the menstrual cup, a trendy option I'd never even heard of before my toxin purge. It works pretty much like a tampon. The silky silicone cup goes up into your baby-shooter and, as you can probably guess from the name, collects the blood until you remove it and pour it out.

At first, the idea of inserting something *all* up in my business had me instinctively clamping my knees together. But the idea intrigued me. Menstrual cups are cost-effective (wash and reuse), clean (no toxins here, baby), and supposedly super comfy (TBD). A survey of more than 1,500 women by menstrual cup maker Intimina found that, compared to using a tampon or wearing a pad, 73 percent reported a boost in comfort while cupping. *Très importante* when cramps are keeping you from kickboxing because 42 percent of women also said that wearing a menstrual cup made them *more likely* to sweat it out during that time of the month.[41]

So I ordered a Lena cup. She arrived all purple and cute. This whole menstrual cup thing couldn't be that bad, right? After giving Lena a boiling bath, I popped her back into her polka dot drawstring pouch until my next period. No sooner had I turned my back than my six-year-old, in all her adorable curiosity, plucked the purple plastic thingy from the bag with her sticky fingers and asked "Mommy, what's this?"

Gah!

"It's something to help Mommy's body, baby."

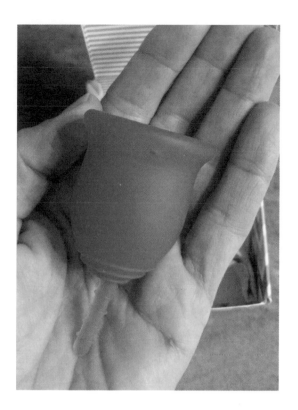

One more bath for Lena and one narrowly avoided period conversation with my still-too-young daughter. Phew.

Sticky fingers aside, if you haven't had kids, this might not be the product for you. My first insertion felt like one part trip to the gyno and one part sex-for-the-first-time awkward. Once things were situated, however, I forgot it was in there, and Lena and I had a flawless leak-free day. Getting it out was . . . messy. After some laborlike ab moves while squatting over the toilet, I delivered little Lena with a splat. The bowl looked like a Jackson Pollock painting. Who knew my V was such an artist?

Bottom line? Lena and I are definitely friends. She's eco-friendly, a great money-saver, and I love that she can hang for up to 12 hours. Unlike Tammy Tampon, she needs no backup and no restocking—just rinse and reinsert. The best part about the cup is that it's totally toxin-free. Definitely worth a try. Happy cupping!

Lena has a ton of gal pals in her girl gang. Other menstrual cup brands available online include:

* Diva Cup
* EvaCup
* Fleur Cup
* Intimina
* Lunette
* Ruby Cup

Congrats! You now have a toxin-free personal care routine, sister! Cue the confetti and razzle dazzle. Now let's take a look at your environment and put all the toxins hiding in your home—in your kitchen cupboards and cleaning supply cabinets—in their rightful place: the trash.

HOUSEHOLD HOSE-DOWN

Mopping always brings out my inner singing Cinderella, but now it's your turn to belt out a cleaner tune. We've made over your body and beauty routine, but the toxins lurking in your household products are worth a look, too. If you wouldn't put these nasty chemicals on your body, you don't want them in the environment where you and your family eat, sleep, and hang out either, right?

In 2015, the International Federation of Gynecology and Obstetrics wrote that "Documented links between prenatal exposure to environmental chemicals and adverse health outcomes span the life course and include impacts on fertility and pregnancy, neurodevelopment, and cancer. The global health and economic burden related to toxic environmental chemicals is in excess of millions of deaths and billions of dollars every year."[42]

That freaky language isn't meant to scare you. Like everything in this book—save my corny jokes—this stuff is both serious and doable. Achieving your healthiest healthy is all about finding the information you need to make the best choices at your own pace so that eventually you can kick those scary statistics to the curb.

The EWG guide rocks here, too. For cleaners, remember they use the A–F rating system, so let's aim for all A's and B's.

Cleaner Cleanup

My hubby often jokes that our kids secretly work for a pest control company. Little crumb trails occur *that* commonly in our home. For our girls, the five-second rule is law. They'll race to grab a stray watermelon ball or a rogue piece of whole wheat mac 'n' cheese that falls onto the counter or floor during meal prep. With these two little scavengers, I seriously stressed about keeping our home in a state of pristine clean. Before earning my honorary degree in personal-care chemistry, that meant eradicating every germy little bugger with a heavy-duty chemical cannon. I holstered up with disinfectant spray and bleach, spraying and scrubbing my way to a spotless shine. Boom!

Then I realized it was time for a research scrub-down. Cleaning supplies contain even more toxins than the pretty potions and tonics we use on our faces. We don't paint our bodies with this yuck, but we're still breathing them in, getting them on our skin, and, in the case of five-second-rule followers, potentially ingesting them. We not only accept heavy-duty germ-fighters, we practically crave them. Cosmetics companies can't use ammonia in their products, but we clean with it like it's no biggie. In this case, we're dealing with a different dictionary of toxins. See pages 92–93 for your cheat sheet.

Rather than scouring my surfaces with these scaries, I scoured blogs and environmental organizations for cleaner alternatives to protect my family without sacrificing my spick-and-span home. You probably already have one of the cleanest

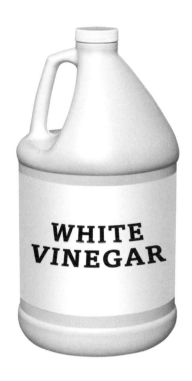

and safest home polishers in your cabinet: distilled white vinegar. This smelly sidekick practically does it all:

* disinfects surfaces
* removes mildew
* declouds glassware
* de-gunks showerheads
* cleans chrome and stainless steel
* refreshes dishwashers and washing machines
* shines windows . . . like the top of the Chrysler Building! (Miss Hannigan would be proud.)

CHEMICALS TO CUT FROM YOUR CLEANING ROUTINE[43]

Ingredient	What It Is	Why It's Harmful
Formaldehyde (formalin)	An industrial-strength disinfectant.	Classified by the World Health Organization as a known human carcinogen.[44]
1,4-dioxane	A manufacturing by-product found in liquid laundry detergent.	Classified by the EPA as a probable human carcinogen.[45]
Bronopol (2-bromo-2-nitropropane-1,3-diol)	Formaldehyde-releasing preservative added to cleaners to help kill bacteria and extend a product's shelf life.	Known to cause negative skin reactions and release low amounts of formaldehyde.[46]
Diethylene glycol monomethyl ether (also known as DEGME, methoxydiglycol)	Found in heavy-duty cleaners, degreasers, and antifreeze.	Linked to fertility issues for women and men, this class of chemicals can be absorbed through the skin or inhaled and reach toxic levels in the body.[47]
Sodium hypochlorite (bleach)	Found in a wide range of cleaners in the laundry room, bathroom, and pool.	An extreme irritant with potent fumes shown to aggravate asthma. Can cause poisoning if inhaled or swallowed.[48]
Ammonium hydroxide	A deep cleaner, degreaser, and polisher used on its own or as an additive.	Ammonia is super corrosive (think chemical burns) and can cause respiratory issues when the fumes are inhaled.[49]

Ingredient	What It Is	Why It's Harmful
Quaternary ammonium compounds: benzalkonium chloride, alkyl dimethyl benzyl ammonium chloride; alkyl dimethyl ethylbenzyl ammonium chloride	These "quats" function as germ busters in antibacterial scrubbers, dish soaps, hand soaps, and disinfecting air fresheners. They also show up in fabric softeners.	Known to cause respiratory issues, including the development or worsening of irritation and asthma.[50]
Ethanolamines (mono-, di-, and triethanolamine)	Used to control acidity in some cleaners; used as detergents in many cleaning products.	Known to cause respiratory issues and irritation.[51]
Perchloroethylene (PCE, PERC)	Used in dry cleaning chemicals, spot cleaners, and polishes, including shoe polish.	According to the National Toxicity Program, this chemical is "reasonably anticipated to be a human carcinogen."[52]
Phthalates	Yep, these scented babies are lurking in your detergents and other cleaning products, too.	Flagged for carcinogenic concerns and reproductive toxicity.[53]

MOTHER NATURE'S CLEANING CABINET

These DIY home-polishers will guarantee a chemical-free sparkle in your home.

Distilled Disinfectant

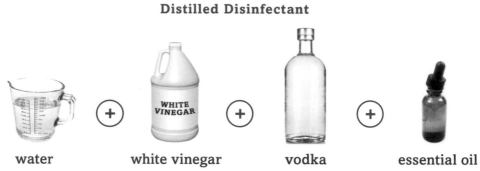

water   **white vinegar**   **vodka**   **essential oil**

In a spray bottle, combine 1½ cups water, ½ cup vinegar, and ½ cup vodka with 20–25 drops essential oil so your house doesn't smell like a bar. Shake to mix.

Shower Shiner

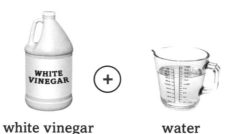

white vinegar   **water**

Mix 4 parts water with 1 part vinegar. Let sit on surfaces 3–5 minutes.

Sink Scrubber/All-Purpose Cleaner

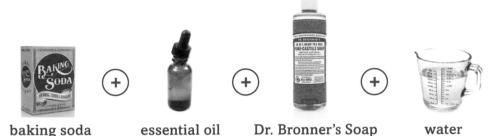

baking soda + **essential oil** + **Dr. Bronner's Soap** + **water**

Mix 1 cup baking soda with 10 drops essential oil. Sprinkle on sink.
Add 1 squirt soap, 3 or 4 drops water, and scrub away.

Streakless Glass Shiner

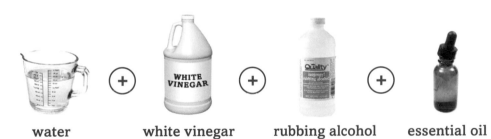

water + **white vinegar** + **rubbing alcohol** + **essential oil**

In a spray bottle, combine 2 cups water, 2 tablespoons vinegar,
2 tablespoons rubbing alcohol, and 2 drops essential oil. Shake and shine.

CLEAN CLEANING SUPPLIES

You don't have to DIY your scrubbers to achieve a cleaner clean. These brands—available online or in select grocery stores—deliver the gleaming countertop goods without all the chemicals.[54]

* AspenClean
* ATTITUDE
* BuggyLOVE
* Dr. Bronner's
* Earth Friendly
* Eco-Me
* ECOS
* Ecover
* Greenshield Organic
* Mrs. Meyers
* Seventh Generation

PLASTICS PURGE

Some plastics are definitely more toxic than others, but they're all a little sketchy. Everything from your yogurt container to the wrap from the deli counter has the potential to leach toxins into your food.[55] Bleh.

In a perfect home, you would go entirely plastic-free in favor of sustainable materials, such as glass and bleach-free paper. In the more likely reality of having some plastics in the house—as we still do—here are the biggies to watch for.

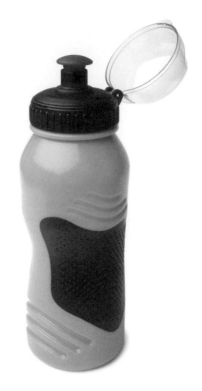

BPAs and Bisphenol-S

Typically added to plastics to make them more durable, like the kind you need in your gym water bottle. These baddies have caught a ton of flack in the media for causing nasty health effects. Like so many items in our makeup, BPA and its cousin bisphenol-S are endocrine disruptors and have been linked to developmental, reproductive, neurological, and immune effects in humans. A 2010 study conducted by researchers at Yale specifically found that prenatal exposure to BPA can increase the risk of breast cancer in the child. Yep, time to bench those BPAs.

Never microwave plastic. Never. Even the self-proclaimed "microwave-safe" kind can leach BPAs and phthalates into your food, and we know what those trashy toxins can do to your body.[56] It's especially likely to happen when you nuke fatty foods, such as meat and cheese. Use microwave-safe glassware or ceramics to cut your exposure to those chemicals.

PVC

The stuff that goes into pipes also goes into lots of different kinds of plastic wrap, including bedding bags and the shrinkwrap in the seafood section. Polyvinyl chloride carries a ton of terrible health risks. Vinyl chloride itself is a human carcinogen, and dioxins released during the manufacturing of PVC can cause reproductive and developmental problems.[57] It also contains endocrine-disrupting phthalates, the same ones linked to breast cancer and reproductive issues.[58] Say sayonara to plastic wrap and, instead, store leftovers in glass containers. If they make it into your grocery bag, no sweat—just ditch the store packaging for your own clean containers as soon as you get home.

Polystyrene

Long story short, using this crunchy white material (brand name: Styrofoam™) can make you seriously sick. Takeout containers and coffee cups can leach styrene—a chemical linked to cancer and nervous system sabotage—especially at high temperatures.[59] Plastic water bottles also contain styrene.[60] Use a ceramic mug to avoid guzzling a side of chemicals with your morning cup of joe and *never* nuke a polystyrene takeout container.

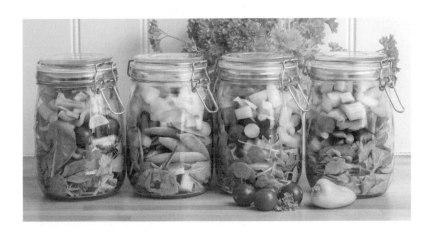

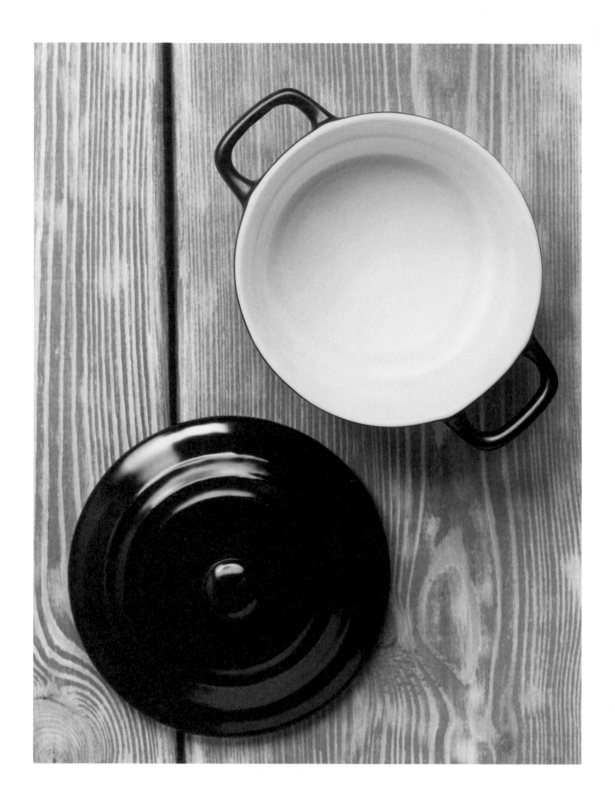

YOUR HEALTHIEST HEALTHY

PFCs

Ever wonder how nonstick coating on pots and pans stands up to heavy-duty heating and all that wacky stuff that infomercials do to prove how scratchproof it is? If you guessed heavy-duty chemicals, *ding ding ding!* Teflon is made from a chemical cocktail called polytetrafluoroetheylene (PTFE), which can release fumes when hanging out over high heat in as few as two minutes. That can give you what scientists call "Teflon flu." Seriously—it can give you flu-like symptoms. The PFC family has been linked to higher cholesterol, liver issues, thyroid trouble, and a compromised immune system.[61] No thanks!

RESULTS!

Time for a progress report. In the first three chapters, you've made HUGE strides toward your healthiest self by making better eating choices, setting healthier goals for your sweat sessions, and trashing your toxic products. Hell-freakin'-yeah, mamacita!

Put this book down and give yourself a pat on the back . . . or booty—go ahead and get crazy. Yes, seriously! Do it! This is BIG stuff, and you're well on your way to living your healthiest healthy ever.

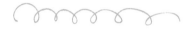

HEALTHY HACK

Unless you want to spend your days and nights scrubbing like Cinderella—instead of just singing like her—you'll need a nonstick alternative. The pros swear that good old-fashioned stainless steel, cast-iron, and ceramic cookware will protect your meal without hindering your chances at earning a Michelin star. PTFE-free red copper or ceramic cookware also does the nonstick job well. If you're stuck with Teflon for now, cook at lower temperatures and switch on the exhaust fan above your stove.

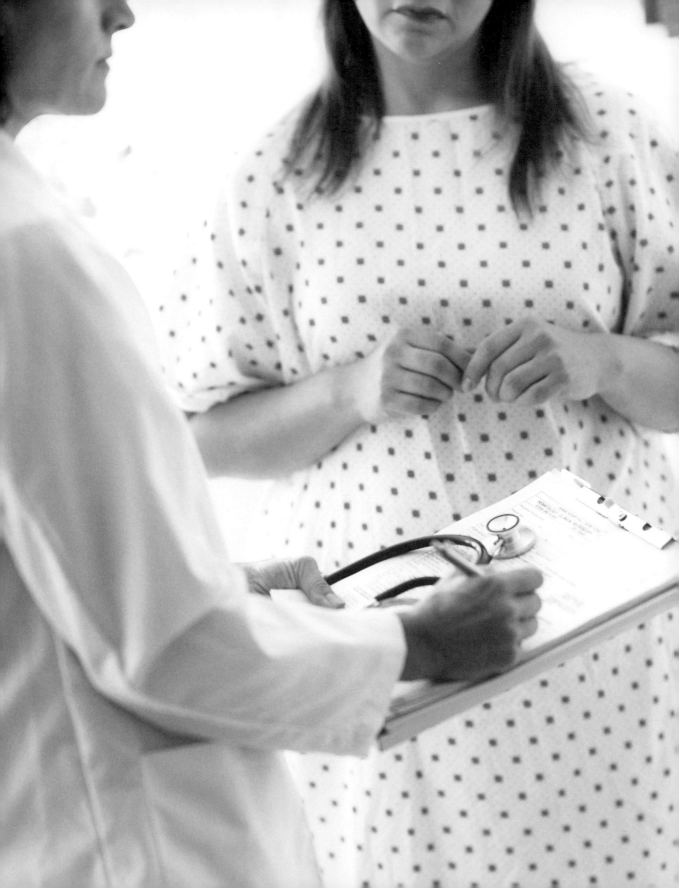

4

MASTER YOUR
MEDICAL MOJO

The C-monster loomed large in my life long before my own lump. When I was 20 years old, my dad received a colon cancer diagnosis. For him, it was a battle. A mover and a doer, he wasn't super vigilant about his health, despite having Crohn's disease. He could have benefited from more of that "medical stuff." Cancer took his life in two short years. He was just 50 years old.

Were his docs not cautious or proactive enough? Did he stick his head in the sand? Either way, by the time they caught his cancer, it was too late—it had metastasized. My daddy put up one hell of a fight, but it's not a fight you want to witness. He taught me many lessons that have made my life infinitely better and more beautiful, but this final example literally saved my life: You can't bury your head in the sand about your health, and you have to have the right pros on your team.

For my father, it was a battle. For me, it was a journey. Vigilance and instinct convinced me early on that something was wrong. People often ask how I knew to push for a better answer about the lump since my mammogram came back with clear results and didn't give me a reason to be looking for issues. Instinct, sure, but nature didn't give me a magical cancer sensor or a medical sixth sense.

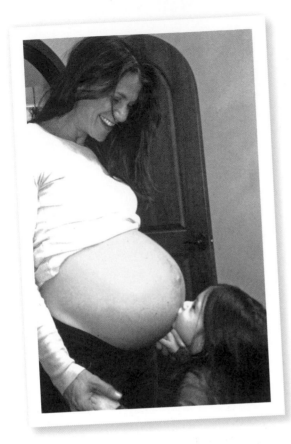

girls—the ones latched and the ones attached—and I got good at it. Feeding my first daughter felt like putting my nips in a vice clamp in the beginning, but eventually I whipped those babies out in the middle of the mall like a sheriff brandishing six-shooters in the Wild West, with nothing but a tiny nursing blankie to cover me. I knew my girls (the ones on my chest) better than the couple of nipple hairs I still have to pluck. (A mastectomy kills the good vibes from boob action, but it doesn't stop the freakin' hair growth? *C'mon!*). By the time I felt the lump, I knew darn well that it hadn't been there before and that I needed to take action. With a team of top docs and my family at my side, treatment and recovery kicked my butt right through to the elusive other side. Count me one of the lucky ones.

In high school and college, I dated more than one musical theater–loving guy who turned out to have zero interest in women. Even my gaydar was off! Years of paying attention to my body and all its processes forged a rock-solid sense of awareness and empowerment about any quirks and warning signs.

Birthing my daughters also made me *way* more comfortable with touching my body than I ever had been. Nursing mothers continually manhandle their

In this chapter, we'll tackle how to get to know your sweet self and increase your awareness of your bod, plus how to assemble the right team of experts who can help you stay vigilant and spring into action when something goes awry. The goal here isn't to turn into you a giant ball of anxiety about your health but to offer you a drawer full of tools to give you a boost of I-got-this confidence . . . and to help you get your head out of the damn sand.

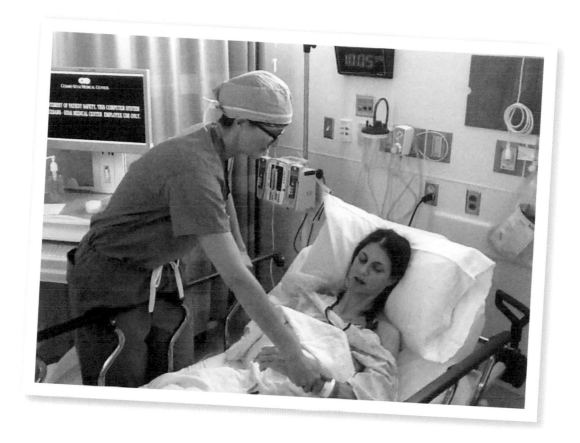

YOUR BODY IQ

How well do you *really* know your bod?

Along with the awareness you can build in the gym, you can learn a lot by paying attention to yourself while gettin' down in the safety of an intimate relationship and through all the beautiful changes you feel during pregnancy and breastfeeding. These experiences will help make you comfortable in your own skin and develop what I call your Body IQ. Think of it like your own personal surveillance system. Your Body IQ consists of two parts:

* a combo of gut feelings and real-life feedback that helps you recognize when something's not right with your health
* the confidence to act on it

No matter how you feel about your bod right now, you can do a lot to get to know it better. Together, we'll shed the mystery (and occasional shame) about how it works to help you develop a solid plan for keeping watch over your well-being. If the idea of getting up close and personal with yourself makes you squirm with a sense of ladylike propriety, no worries: You don't have to be an exhibitionist about your poop or blemishes. It's totally fine to share those details solely with your docs. Either way, though, you should explore your body with curiosity, respect, and gratitude for all the amazing things it can do!

Get to Know Your Girls

Kids or no kids, breastfeeding or formula, it doesn't matter. Get to know those ta-tas pronto. Experts say the best time for a breast self-exam is five to seven days after your period starts, when your ladies tend to feel less tender and lumpy.[1] Yes ma'am, you gotta grab those babies monthly!

BREAST SELF-EXAM IN FOUR EASY STEPS

After a long day, I like to release my lady lumps from their boulder holder and circle them around a bit in their own soft tissue soft shoe—side to side, back and forth, *five, six, seven, eight!* This little boob dance helped me find that abnormal clump of cells. Don't be afraid to fondle daily and note any changes. If you prefer to stick to a more traditional check, here's how.[2]

STEP 1 Strip down and stand in front of a mirror. *Hey there, hot stuff!* Keep your shoulders straight and put your hands on your hips, Wonder Woman–style. Here's what you're looking for:

* changes in the size, shape, or color of your breasts
* skin that looks dimply, puckered, indented, or scaly
* changes in the position or direction of your nipples (an outie suddenly becoming an innie)
* rashes, redness, or swelling
* nipple discharge that looks milky, watery, yellow, or red

On that last point, it's totally normal to ooze milk if you're breastfeeding—not so much if your youngest just graduated from high school.

STEP 2 Repeat with your arms raised.

STEP 3 Time to feel yourself up! Lie down on a flat surface, which gives you the best angle on all the breast tissue. Put one hand behind your head and use the first few finger pads of the opposite hand—left hand on right boob, right hand on left boob—to make quarter-size circles. Either start at the nipple and move outward, or work up and down in vertical lines, whichever way you prefer, but make sure you handle your *entire* breast. Here's what you're feeling for:

* lumps
* pain or soreness
* thick or firm tissue
* anything different from your normal

Breast Self-Examination

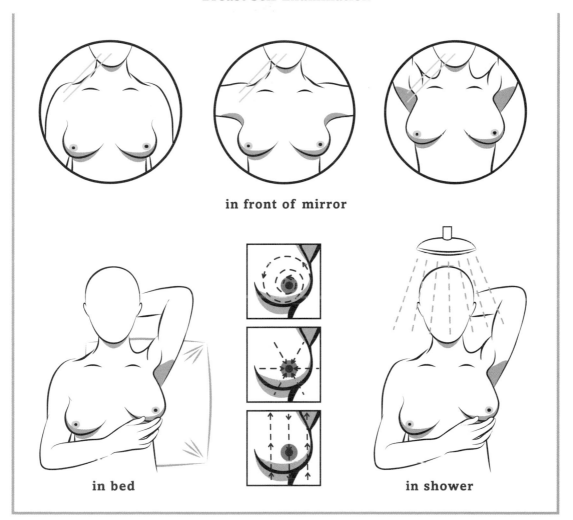

in front of mirror

in bed

in shower

STEP 4 Repeat while standing or sitting to make double sure you've inspected every inch. Pro tip: Getting soaped up in the shower will help you feel if something's not right. Don't forget to feel around your pits for any lumps, too.

If you find something strange, don't panic. Call a breast specialist or ask your regular doc for a referral. Best to have it checked by someone who examines breasts all day rather than relying on the more generalized skills of your regular doc—as I did for months. Odds are high that it's *not* cancer. Your monthly cycle, hormonal fluctuations, breastfeeding, and other events can cause temporary changes in your breasts.

In the rare case that you find yourself in my shoes, stay calm. We'll deal with accepting and breaking the news, one step at a time, in chapter 5.

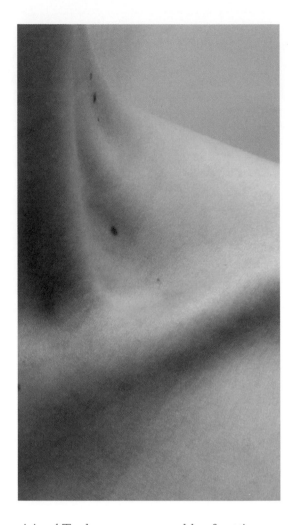

MAP YOUR MOLES

Your skin changes faster than your feelings about kale. It regenerates in about a month.[3] That process helps protect your insides with a self-repairing coat of armor—anyone else feel like a warrior princess?—but those rapidly dividing cells also create the perfect environment for cancer to thrive.

Skin cancer is the most common kind of cancer, and incidents of melanoma, the most deadly type of skin cancer, are rising.[4] To decrease your odds of getting it, stay away from the tanning salon. My grandparents had a freakin' tanning bed in their house, so mole checks top my list. Reign supreme as a sunscreen queen—even in winter and on cloudy days. Remember, though, that still doesn't make your skin cancer-proof.

You can spot the most common signs: a new growth, a sore that doesn't heal, or a change in the color or shape of a mole or mark. Every six months to a year, get a full once-over by a pro—even in the places where the sun don't shine!—and keep tabs on yourself every month or two to become familiar with your beauty marks, blemishes, freckles, and moles. You're most likely to notice any potentially concerning changes, but it doesn't hurt to recruit the help of your partner. Hey, if you do them right, skin checks can be sexy!

HEALTHY HACK

Some derms have fancy mole-mapping software, which is super cool. If yours doesn't, you can DIY. Snap photos of your moles with your phone and file them in a program like Evernote. Make sure to record dates and locations since close-ups can make it hard to tell whether that's the bend in your elbow or your booty crack! This hack gives you a historical record for time-lapse comparisons, and it makes it easy peasy to show your dermatologist.

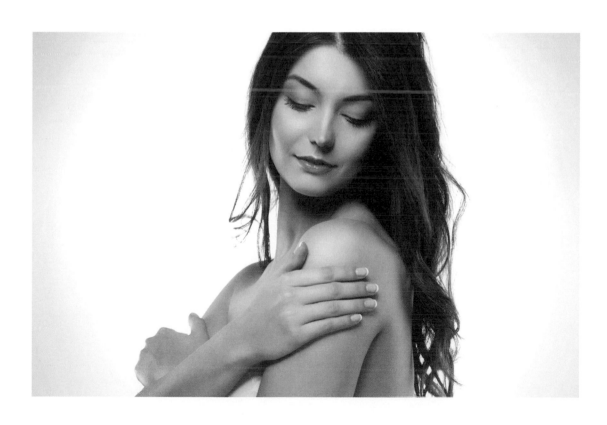

FIVE-STEP SKIN CHECK

Follow these five simple steps from the experts at the American Academy of Dermatology to keep tabs on your skin.[5]

1. Get naked and give your sexy self a good once-over in the mirror—front and back—especially your legs. Don't forget to hike up your boobs so you can get a look underneath. While you're at it, why not kill two birds and do your breast exam?

2. Bend your elbows to scope out your forearms, then your palms. Make sure to look at the backs of your upper arms. If everything looks OK, flex and admire those triceps!

3. Sit down and focus on your feet, including your soles, the spaces between your toes, and underneath your toenails. Skin cancer can appear as a thick dark line under your nail. If you love a good pedi, make sure to sneak a good peek at your bare nails between polish changes.

4. Grab a hand mirror and check the back of your neck and scalp. Use a blow dryer to help move hair out of the way so you can see your entire noggin.

5. With the hand mirror, also check your back, bum, and lady parts. Yep, skin cancer can strike you even there!

As you do, follow the A-B-C-D-E of skin cancer concerns.[6]

* **A**symmetry—Half the mole or mark doesn't look the same as the other half.
* **B**order—Edges look jagged, scalloped like your grandma's doily, or otherwise uneven.
* **C**olor—Rather than a single shade of brown, the mole is multicolored, and may even turn black, red, white, or blue. Not a good way to show your patriotism!
* **D**iameter—Is it bigger than a quarter of an inch? That's 6 millimeters for my metric friends, or about the size of a pencil eraser. Some melanomas are smaller, but bigger doesn't mean better in this case.
* **E**volving—Your skin changes over time, but is it changing faster than other similar spots?

Again, if you find something strange, don't freak. Document it and get to the derm for a professional look.

ODE DE TOILET

In middle school, one of my best friends—name withheld to protect the guilty—and I made up a whole series of tunes about going number two. Size, shape, the whole smelly process of getting it from body to bowl—oh, yeah, we sang about our poop. I haven't the faintest idea what inspired our little shit shows (pun totally intended), but we thought we were downright hilarious. Years of embarrassment later, it turns out we were on to something.

You don't have to croon about your crap, but you should pay enough attention to bathroom behaviors to be able to jot down a few notes, if not a whole chorus. Your poop, in particular, can prove super valuable when it comes to surveying your health.[7] At the very least, you should peek before flushing the evidence. If what you see looks at all unusual, make a note to discuss it with your doctor. Those conversations may feel uncomfortable, but they can shed light on your overall digestive wellness as well as more serious intestinal issues.

Everyone's poop varies, and yours may shift based on diet, illness, and medications. In other words, don't automatically assume the worst, says Dr. Niket Sonpal, a gastroenterologist and professor of medicine in New York City. If anything seems out of the ordinary for more than a few days, tell your doc.

HEALTHY HACK

Exercise, hydration, and a fiber-rich diet all help keep you on a regular schedule. If you have to strain hard to drop the kids off at the pool or you have ongoing belly bloat, possibly due to backed-up bowels, here are two ways to help get things moving.

Give yourself a colon massage. Gently rub from the lower right side of your belly to the upper right side (ascending colon). Then knead it from right to left, about two inches below your belly button, moving across (transverse colon) and down to the lower left of your abdomen (descending colon).

A poop stool, such as the Squatty Potty, that elevates your feet while you do your business may help because it straightens the angle of the rectal canal, which can move things along as well.

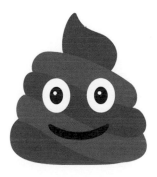

WHAT YOUR POO IS TELLING YOU

Once you start paying attention to your poop, you may need to doo-doo diligence. Here are some of the most common changes to your digestive leftovers, what might be causing them, and when you might have cause for concern.

Color

Fifty Shades of Brown is fair game for your healthy norm. Here's what other shades might be saying.[8]

Color	Potential Cause	When to Worry
Green	Green gut remnants can occur when stool moves too fast through your intestines—such as when you have diarrhea—or when you eat a ton of green leafy veggies.	You don't have the runs or haven't eaten lots of greens.
White	Chalky crapola sometimes results from medications such as Pepto Bismol, but it also can indicate a bile duct obstruction.	You haven't had indigestion.
Yellow	Unless you're a breastfed newborn, this shade can happen because of a digestive issue, such as gluten sensitivity. It's usually extra stinky and may appear to have a greasy texture.	You don't have a history of gluten issues.
Black	Gobbling black licorice or taking iron supplements sometimes causes black in the bowl. It also could mean blood in your stool—not good.	You haven't started taking iron supplements or eaten lots of black food.
Red	Harmless dietary changes—eating beets or chugging red sports drinks—can be a red herring . . . or you might have intestinal bleeding.	You haven't eaten anything red.
Turquoise	That time when my daughters ate an ocean-themed cake with excessive food coloring.	Right away . . . until remembering that crazy birthday cake!

Bristol Stool Chart

	Type 1	Separate hard lumps	severe constipation
	Type 2	Lumpy and sausagelike	mild constipation
	Type 3	A sausage shape with cracks in the surface	normal
	Type 4	Like a smooth, soft sausage or snake	normal
	Type 5	Soft blobs with clear-cut edges	lacking fiber
	Type 6	Mushy consistency with ragged edges	mild diarrhea
	Type 7	Liquid consistency with no solid pieces	severe diarrhea

Shape & Size

"The size of stool varies by the amount of fiber that you eat—the more bulk, the bigger the poops are," says Dr. Sonpal. The Bristol Stool Chart officially recognizes seven types of stool, but you want to fall between 3 and 5. Type 4 is considered the perfect poo. If your stool is too soft or too hard, you probably need to Goldilocks your diet. Bust out that food journal and then talk to your doc about what you're eating.[9]

Smell

Don't act like your stuff don't stank; everyone's does. But unbearably stinky stool or something seriously unusual might signal an issue such as Crohn's disease or celiac disease.[10]

Buoyancy

Dietary changes—namely noshing on insoluble fibers such as bran or starch—are the top reason your poop might float. Along with artificial sweeteners, these foods can cause gas, which pumps your poo full of extra air. Lactose intolerance and gluten sensitivity can have the same effect, says Dr. Sonpal.

Frequency

"When we talk about regularity, what we're really talking about is what's regular for *you*," says Dr. Sonpal. Depending on what you eat and how often, anything from three times a day to three times a week is considered healthy.

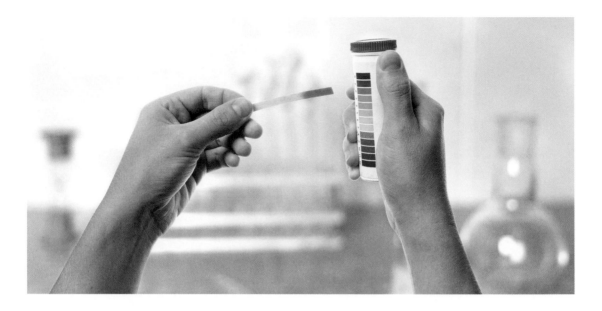

FREE TO PEE, YOU AND ME

Score some more major Body IQ points by keeping tabs on the pH of your pee. If you need a quick refresher from high school chem, "pH" refers to how acidic or basic something is. The pH scale runs from 1 to 14. The low end indicates something acidic, 7 is perfectly neutral, and the high end points to basic or alkaline substances.[11]

A pH-balanced bod keeps good and bad bacteria in balance, staves off unwanted inflammation, and wards off weight gain for optimal health.[12] An out-of-whack pH reading for your pee can signal gastric issues, kidney problems, or a urinary tract infection (UTI).[13]

pH Scale

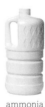

ammonia

| 0 | 1 | 2 | 3 | 4 | 5 | 6 | 7 | 8 | 9 | 10 | 11 | 12 | 13 | 14 |

ACIDIC   NEUTRAL   ALKALINE

To check the pH of your pee:

* Order some inexpensive urine pH test strips, which you can find online or at most drugstores.
* Test your second tinkle of the day, when any accumulated acidity has started to disperse.
* Slip that strip in your stream and wait for the results.

So what's normal? Well, your pee changes throughout the day. It starts slightly more acidic in the morning, and it becomes more alkaline as your body digests food.[14] Mainly diet affects your pH balance. Eating more leafy greens, beans, and seeds, and reducing your consumption of animal protein, coffee, cheese, and alcohol will keep you in the pHerfect range.

Don't worry if a reading or two look out of line. Minor shifts in your diet and other habits can throw you off temporarily.[15] Track your levels over time and talk to your health care team if it's consistently too low (more likely), too high, or changing considerably.

HEALTHY HACK

If slipping a strip into your stream makes you scream, spit into a cup and test your saliva instead.

LYMPH LESSONS

Time for a pop quiz!

QUIZ

True or false?

All of your vital fluids travel through your bloodstream.
❏ True ❏ False

If you said true, let me introduce you to the lymphatic system.

You know those glands in your neck that can swell up when you're sick, giving you a super-hot double chin? They also show up in a lot of cancer cases. During my mastectomy, my doctors discovered that the cancer had spread to a lymph node in my armpit, so they removed that and all the surrounding nodes to be safe. People with fewer lymph nodes have a lifetime risk of lymphedema, a permanent swelling of the limbs (way uncomfy and with its own set of issues), so lymphatic system checkups have become a regular part of my health care routine.

People with what experts call "intact" lymph nodes don't need to exert quite as much vigilance about this issue, but everyone can benefit from knowing about the lymphatic system and how to show it more love. To break it down for you, here's my own lymphatic specialist, Lisa Levitt Gainsley, a certified lymphedema therapist: "The lymphatic system—part of your immune system—is the body's great recycling system. Lymphatic fluid moves like rivers through your body, transporting excess waste and toxins to the lymph nodes. There, white blood cells, macrophages, and lymphocytes filter out the waste and return clean lymphatic fluid to your bloodstream. Unlike the blood, the lymphatic system doesn't have a central pump. It depends on muscle movement and is optimized by manual lymphatic drainage (MLD). Among other benefits, MLD reduces inflammation, softens scar tissue, alleviates side effects of cancer treatment, manages lymphedema, and speeds up recovery after surgery. MLD is a soothing treatment, which relaxes the nervous system and brings the body to the parasympathetic state where healing occurs."

Loving your lymph nodes with a little extra TLC (tender lymphatic care), outlined below, can help your body remove toxins, boost digestive function, and leave you feeling lighter and more refreshed.

* **Get a Lymphatic Massage.** More spas and wellness centers are offering lymphatic massages, which focus on your nodes and keep the system flowing the way it should. If you have or have had cancer or lack some lymph nodes for any reason, make sure the therapist has a certification in rerouting the fluid. Search for qualified professionals at lymphnet.org.

* **Keep up with your gym routine.** The best exercises for your lymphatic system include swimming—because the water pressure helps move the fluid through your body—and rebounding on a mini trampoline. If you have kiddos who want to join the fun, go for a full-size trampoline.

Lymphatic dry-brushing paths and points

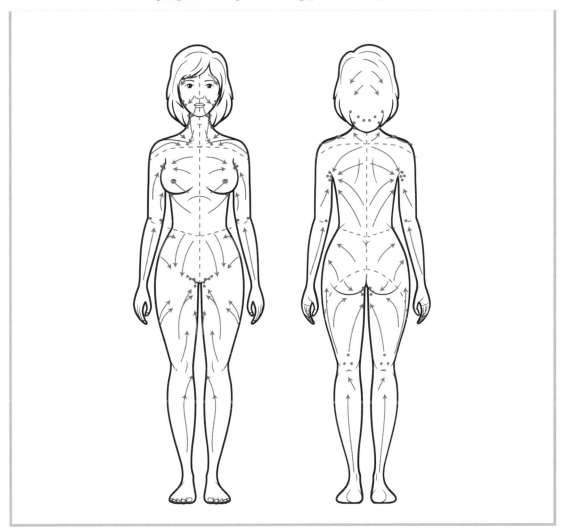

* **Cut the crap**—from your diet, that is. Follow an anti-inflammatory diet, like the one we discussed in chapter 1, that also limits salt and alcohol for peak lymph health.

* **Dry-brush yourself.** This involves moving a long-handled brush with soft, natural bristles over your skin. The trick is to brush in the direction that your lymph fluid flows. Check out some online videos to help you master the technique.

KNOW YOUR NUMBERS

To develop a solid Body IQ, you gotta know your numbers! That involves keeping track of a *lot* of important health stats, but you don't have to go to med school to know what's healthy. Use the handy chart below, which covers the most important figures to track. For

Test	What's Normal?	What Happens If You're Not?
Blood pressure[16]	**< 120/80 mm/Hg** 120–139 systolic (first number) and/or 80–89 diastolic (second number) is considered pre-hypertension. **140+ systolic (first number) or 90+ diastolic (second number) officially puts you in the high blood pressure zone.**[17]	High blood pressure can hurt your heart, kidneys, eyes, and nearly every other organ in your body. But you can take lots of steps to control it! Your doc might advise exercise, changes in diet, or medication.
Cholesterol[18]	**< 200 mg/dL, the lower the better** 200–239 **240+**	High cholesterol blocks your arteries and harms your heart. As with blood pressure, healthy habits can help bring it under control. Again, in certain cases, your doc might recommend meds to treat it, but, no matter what, a healthy diet as described in chapter 1 is essential.
Body fat percentage[19]	**<15 percent** 15–19 percent **20–24 percent** 25–32 percent **33+ percent verges on obesity** (These percentages refer to women.)	Body mass index (BMI) assessments measure the ratio of your height to your weight, so that measurement classifies a lot of super fit people as obese because muscle is denser than fat. Dumb. Body fat percentage offers a much more accurate measure of health because it pays attention to your body composition. Even if you fit into your skinny jeans, you could be storing too much fat, which increases your odds of developing heart disease, diabetes, cancer, etc. If your body fat percentage is too low, you can have bone, hormone, and other problems. Talk to your doc about gaining weight safely because bingeing on cheeseburgers isn't part of that protocol.

each measure, check whether you fall into the healthy range and, if you don't, ask your doc what you can do to get back on track.

Test	What's Normal?	What Happens If You're Not?
Waist circumference[20]	**<35 inches** **35+** (If you can pinch more than an inch of fat near your belly button, you are at increased risk for cardiovascular disease.)	Some research suggests this number is even more important than BMI because belly fat poses a bigger threat to cardiovascular health than fat elsewhere in your body. Shrink your waist by mixing up your workouts to include strength training and cardio and steer clear of simple, sugary carbs in your diet.
Blood sugar[21]	**< 99 mg/dL** 100–125 is the prediabetes zone **126+ qualifies you for a diabetes diagnosis** (Doctors use a few different tests to measure blood sugar; these numbers reference the results of a fasting plasma glucose test. Ask which test you're getting and what the numbers mean.)	Type 2 diabetes harms your heart and other aspects of your health. Again, a healthy diet—limiting sugary, simple carbs and processed foods—and exercise pay off.

Now that you've boosted your Body IQ by knowing your health stats and what they mean, do a celebratory shimmy-shimmy-booty-shake. Woohoo! The next step is learning how to use that info with the pros to get your medical mojo into its healthiest groove ever.

STANDARDIZED TEST PREP

A mammogram fewer than two weeks before I found my lump missed my breast cancer completely, but expert-recommended tests for cancer and other diseases really do play a key role in keeping us healthy. Regular checks can

spot health problems early, when they're easiest to treat.

At the same time, you don't want to go overboard. Who wants to live at the doctor's office? In your 20s, start doing regular breast self-exams and skin checks, per the guidelines in this chapter. Keep up that savvy body behavior until your ta-tas are sagging and your skin becomes a proud collection of laugh lines. Apart from that, there's no one-size-fits-all pu-pu platter for health tests. It's all about personalization based on your unique risk factors. The table at the right gives you a cheat sheet for which tests to take at what age and when.

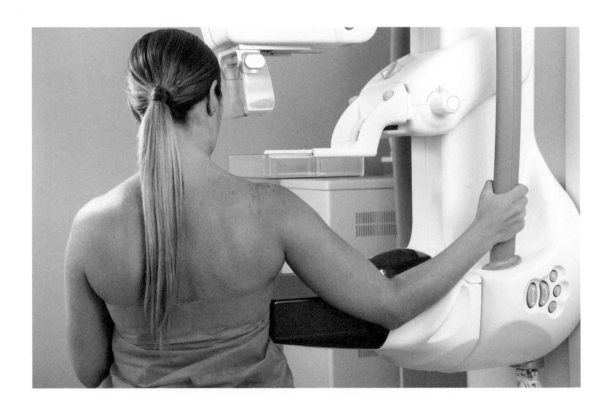

Age	Test	When
20s **Keep getting these four tests into the next decade and beyond.**	Pap smear[22]	Every 3 years
	Breast exam	Have your gyno give the girls a look once a year in addition to your monthly self-checks.
	Blood pressure test[23]	Every 2 years. If you have a family history of heart issues, make it yearly.
	Cholesterol test[24]	Every 4–6 years
30s	Thyroid test[25]	At age 35 and every 5 years afterward, this test can tell you if any funky hormones are affecting your organs.
	Glaucoma test[26]	Every 2–4 years. At age 40, up the frequency to every 1–3 years. In your 50s, every 1–2 years. In your 60s, every 6 months.
40s	Mammogram[27]	Starting at age 40, schedule a regular boob smoosh every 1–2 years. Make it 3D if available to you.
	Diabetes screening[28]	Starting at age 45, every 2 years
	Blood pressure[29]	Every year
50s	Colonoscopy[30]	Every 10 years. If you have risk factors, ask your doctor how often you need to take this test. Think of the prep as a wellness retreat–like colonic.
60s	Bone density[31]	Starting at age 65, every 1–2 years

As a general rule, if you have a family history of anything, start getting screened *earlier* than someone who doesn't. If you have additional risk factors, here's how to customize your screening schedule.

* **Breast cancer:** If you have a family history, start your screenings 10 years before the age at which your relative was diagnosed. Other risk factors include BRCA gene mutations or a personal history of breast cancer.[32]

* **Cholesterol:** If you smoke, have diabetes, or have a family history of heart disease, start cholesterol checks in your 20s.[33]

* **Colorectal cancer:** Family history, a diet high in red meats or alcohol, weight issues, smoking, and type 2 diabetes all increase risk. People of African or European Jewish descent may also have a higher risk.[34]

* **Glaucoma:** Subpar vision, poor circulation, diabetes, and migraines are all risk factors. People of African and Hispanic heritage should consider earlier, more frequent screenings.[35]

* **Osteoporosis:** Family history, low body weight, and a personal history of fractures put you at increased risk. Caucasian and Asian women are at particularly high risk.[36]

* **Skin cancer:** Family history, blistering sunburns as a kid or teen, fair skin, a track record of indoor tanning (guilty!), and many moles warrant earlier, more frequent skin checks. Blondes and redheads also should pay closer attention.[37]

* **Thyroid:** Family history of thyroid conditions warrants starting those tests at age 20. Get tested right away if you're showing any signs for hypothyroidism (constipation, dry skin, fatigue, sensitivity to cold, and unexplained weight gain).[38]

* **Type 2 diabetes:** Being overweight in childhood or adulthood can increase your risk of developing the disease, as can inactivity and high blood pressure. People of Native American, African, Hispanic, and Asian/South Pacific Islander descent also have a higher risk. Women with polycystic ovarian syndrome also have a higher risk.[39]

In the earliest days of my healthiest healthy journey, I determined to find out everything possible about my cancer and what might have caused it. I had genetic tests and blood tests galore. It turned out that I didn't have any hereditary biomarkers that predisposed me for cancer. Part relief because my little angels likely won't have them either, part frustrating because why the eff had this happened to me? Those tests taught me a lot about my health and how to take it to the next level.

Blood Tests

We could spend an entire book talking about what you can learn from a blood test, so the best way to figure out which blood tests you should take is to talk to your doctor about your unique health sitch. Because mama loves her sushi, I have my mercury levels tested two or three times a year as well as my levels of vitamin D, iron, zinc, cholesterol, blood cell counts, etc. I'm over the age of 35, so I also get regular blood tests to check my thyroid levels.

Genetic Tests

Body-savvy tech can tell you more than ever about your body's past, present, and future. A simple spit swab can reveal your predisposition to diseases, possible degenerative issues such as hair or hearing loss, and your fitness potential (likely muscle composition, speed, endurance, and more). When you want to learn more about how your body works at a cellular level and what might be hiding in your DNA, genetic tests can be lifesavers—literally.

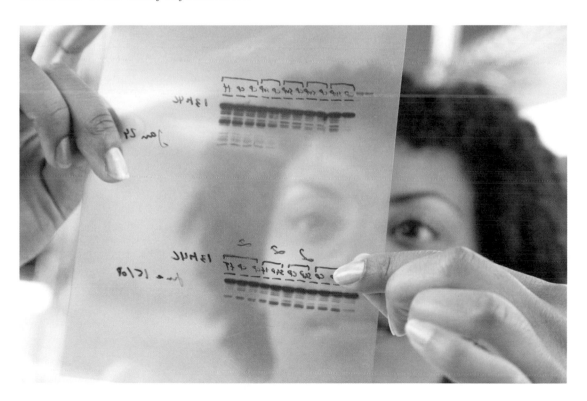

ROCK YOUR DOC SQUAD

There's a lot you can do in your daily life to find your healthiest healthy, and you also can benefit from the expertise of the pros. That's why *they* pulled the all-nighters in med school. In this section, let's put that Body IQ to good use to build a top-notch team of experts, the support squad ready to rappel in, *Mission Impossible*–style, at a moment's notice! Here's how to assemble your crew(s)—Tom Cruise not included.

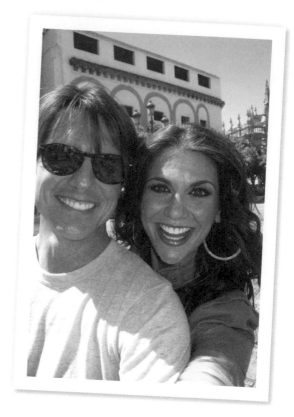

In my healthiest healthy, I have a deep doctor bench, including physicians who practice both Western medicine and alternative modalities. With so many specialists, it's like shopping for good health. Just like going wild at Bloomies, shopping for a doc squad can require serious cash. Unfortunately, comprehensive health care isn't a given for many people. Ridiculous, isn't it? In the entertainment industry, where freelance employment status is the norm, I lost my insurance between my lumpectomy and my mastectomy. Scary! Thankfully and luckily I reobtained it through my husband's job.

Even with continuous coverage, money sometimes prevents people from getting the health care they want or need. My insurance doesn't cover my lymphatic drainage therapist, for instance. Seeing a dozen doctors isn't always an option, so here's how to break your doc squad down into levels, from the essential basics to the ultimate specialists. When your budget allows or you definitely have a specific medical issue, level up. It's worth it.

Of course, quality totally trumps quantity when it comes to stacking your team. Same goes with expertise over bells and whistles. Give points for your doc's big-ass brain and on-point patient skills, not her designer shoes, fancy waiting room, complimentary coffee bar, or impeccable makeup.

Must Have
primary care physician, dentist, optometrist

No ifs, ands, or buts about it, you must have someone who can see you right away in an emergency and check you out yearly to screen for red flags. Even if you don't wear glasses or need help with your smile, you must have your eyes and teeth checked regularly.

Should Have
gynecologist, dermatologist

Every gal needs a gyno, period. In a pinch, your primary care physician can help monitor any private-part problems, but you really should have someone whose sole job is to look at vaginas. Same goes for skin.

Nice to Have
integrative internist, chiropractor, massage therapist

For holistic health, an integrative practitioner or a functional medicine doc can give you the most comprehensive care. Beyond that, everyone can benefit from a team of experts trained in helping you get your body right—especially after hard-core gym sessions.

Really Nice to Have
specialists

In a perfect world, cap your doc squad with specialists in every field: gastroenterologist, breast specialist, podiatrist, physical therapist, and more. Prioritize what's most important for your health. If you have a family history of colon cancer, definitely enlist the services of a gastroenterologist.

Any Health Care Provider

Look for doctors who check their egos at the door and take the time to educate you as the patient, whether that means explaining step by step what's going on in your body or giving you practical tools and techniques that you can use when you're not in their office. An informed and educated patient is an empowered patient!

Primary Care Physician

This relationship is likely to be long-term, so look for a stellar resume and a compatible personality. "You want to find a doctor who seems engaged in caring for you and who actually *likes* being a doctor," says Dr. Delia Chiaramonte, associate director and director of education at the Center for Integrative Medicine at the University of Maryland School of Medicine. "Burned-out doctors have patients who have worse outcomes." Look for someone who really loves what he or she does.

Specialist

"This is not the time to choose for convenience. You want the most highly trained person for what you need them to do," says Dr. Darria Long Gillespie, senior vice president of clinical strategy at Sharecare and a national media expert who helps women and children live healthier lives. "You want someone

who has seen a thousand people before you and has seen every permutation of complexity." If you need a procedure, look for someone who's done it at least a hundred times. If it's a rare procedure, you want the person who has done it more than anyone else in your region. Remember, the most famous doctor might not always be the most skilled. Sometimes the most up-to-date physician is one of the junior members of the staff.

With a dozen different "docs" buzzing in an out of the room, you might find it hard to keep track of who's treating you. "I see many patients confused by the different titles, since many medical professionals (nurses, PAs, lab techs) now wear white coats," says Dr. Gillespie. "If in doubt, it's always OK to ask if someone is a physician and, if not, what his or her title is. You always have the right to know who is providing your care."

HEALTHY HACK

Don't be afraid to "date" your doc. If you don't get great vibes after a visit or two, go ahead and ghost.

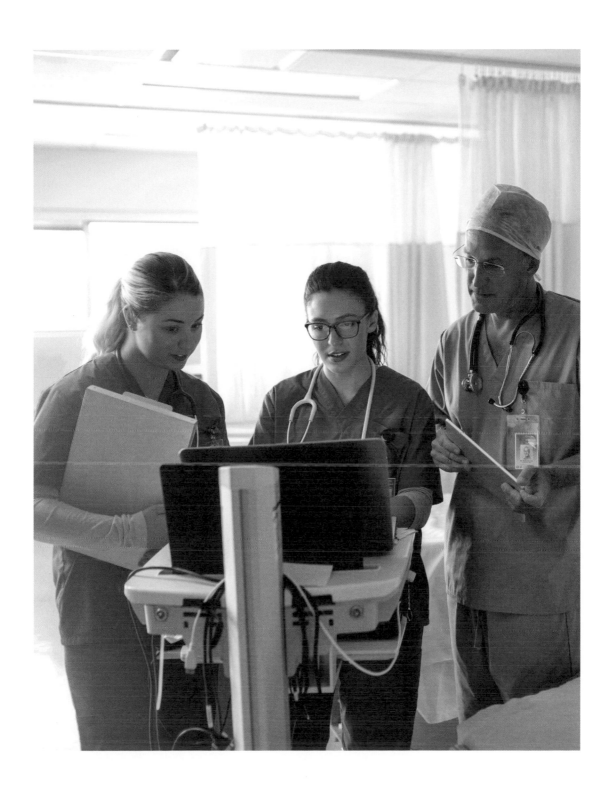

HOW TO TALK TO YOUR DOC

Put on your journalist hat and let's look at the questions to ask your doctor.

When You're "Doc Dating"

No, not like *that*—though if you are dating a doctor, good for you! No, I mean those early days of courting a new doctor to see if he or she is the right fit for you.

* How do you approach patient education? How does that fit into patient care?
* In terms of treatments and care, how do you stay current on the latest research? How will that inform my care?
* How will you make use of your medical peers to determine advice for me?
* How digitally connected is your practice? Can I check my charts online or with an app?
* How much do you integrate nontraditional approaches into your treatment?
* What's the best way to communicate with you if I need answers fast or in an emergency?

When You're Healthy

Just because all your tests have come out A-OK and all your numbers are living happily in the green zone doesn't mean you shouldn't stay engaged during your exam.

* How does my health compare to the last time I was in the office? Are there any changes (dietary or otherwise) that I should consider making?
* Should I start seeing a specialist based on anything in my family history or current health profile?
* Which screenings would you recommend, based on my age, gender, ethnicity, or health risks?
* What's the number one thing I can do to improve my health?

After Receiving a Diagnosis

Don't be afraid to ask your doc whom else you should speak to. Again, a good doctor will check his or her ego at the door.

* If you had just received this diagnosis, who would you go to for care?
* If I were your daughter, mother, or sister, what course of treatment would you recommend?
* Which resources and websites should I use to find more info about this?
* Should I see any other specialists?
* What can I expect in the next two weeks? The next month? Six months from now? A year from now?
* How can I best prepare myself for what's to come?
* Is there any palliative care available to me?

During Recovery

You're out of the woods, but that doesn't mean you and your doc are never ever getting back together (catchy Taylor Swift references courtesy of my music-loving daughters). You need to stay in touch.

* How long is the recovery process? If I'm still experiencing pain or fatigue after that window, what should I do?
* What complications or warning signs warrant a call to you? What about a trip to the emergency room?
* What nutrition and activity changes do I need to make during the recovery period?
* How soon will I be able to get back to my regular daily activities?
* What additional specialists should I see to promote my recovery?
* What can I do to keep this from happening again in the future?

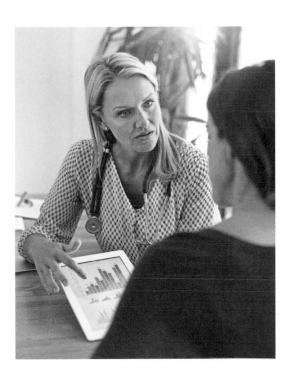

HEALTHY HACK

If at any point you don't understand something your doc is saying, ask her to phrase it differently, be more specific, speak more simply, or even draw a picture. Her job is to make sure *you* understand all the information, so never feel afraid or embarrassed to speak up!

DECODING DOC TALK

Docs routinely rattle off results that don't make sense to us laypeople before recording them in a mysterious digital chart that floats off into cyberspace. Then, in a flash, they fly out of the exam room. *Sheesh!*

I didn't study "doctor" as my foreign language in school, but I did talk to a *lot* of them while assembling my healthiest health squad. You can decode all that jargon à la Nancy Drew, learn to ask the right questions, and achieve waiting room A-list status by becoming the best, most informed patient you can be. Let's put that Body IQ to the test.

Office Visit Action Plan

Before	* Keep track of any symptoms you have, such as pain, stomachaches, sleeplessness, low energy, new growths, or unusual bleeding, using your phone or a good old pen and paper. Include when they started and what makes them better or worse. * List all the medications you take. Absolutely everything. This includes over-the-counter drugs and supplements—yep, even your daily vitamin C gummy. Your doc needs to know what you're taking in case of allergic reaction or medicinal combos that don't mix well (contraindications). If it helps you keep track, gather the bottles together and snap a photo before you leave the house. * Write down your questions and concerns in descending order of importance so you remember them in the heat of the moment. This will help you stay focused in the presence of Dr. Rush-more. Remember, she's there for you!
During	* Always take notes. If it's an important visit—say, you're discussing test results—you might even bring a friend or relative to help or ask if you can record the convo so you don't miss any of the important deets. * Be totally honest, no matter what. One survey found that nearly a third of women lie to their docs about everything: how much they exercise, what they eat, their sex lives, and more.[40] Bad idea! Your doc needs the full truth—drunken nights, poor life decisions, and all. Fibbing only hurts you. * Understand everything the doc says. Don't let him or her out the door until you do and you know your next steps. Ask as many questions as you need to ask.
After	* Follow up to get test results and updates. If you're expecting to hear from your doctor, keep checking in until you get answers. * Ask for copies of your medical records and keep them in a folder, either online or off. * Contact your doctor or other health care pros, such as nurses or pharmacists, if you have new symptoms or questions about your health or treatments.

Bottom line: You are the ultimate authority on your body. Learn all about your bod's systems, its processes and rhythms, and follow your gut when things don't feel right, and you'll be on your way to your healthiest healthy faster than a doc can dash from an exam room.

Not only will staying tuned into your body have a huge impact on your health, but it also may save you some cash. Research shows that engaged patients—those who take an active role in their wellness and medical care—have healthier lives and lower medical costs in the long run.[41] Doesn't a new pair of killer heels seem like a better place to sink your cash than easily preventable doctor visits? Even better, make it a new pair of running shoes!

As a busy working mom, I get it. Just making it to that annual checkup or gyno appointment—let alone prepping before and following up after—feels like a feat. But don't deprioritize looking out for *your* best health while you're looking out for everyone else. Spending a little time to organize yourself can make a big difference in how much you get out of those few minutes of one-on-one time with your MD. The more you take care of yourself, the more you will be around and able to take care of everyone else.

Now let's put a shiny gold star of accomplishment on part one of this book! We've covered a *whole lotta* information about your body and how it operates best: what you put in it, how you keep it running, what you put on and around it, and how to listen up and call in expert reinforcements when needed.

But please, *pretty please*, don't feel overwhelmed that you aren't doing every single thing we've discussed so far. This didn't all happen overnight for me, and it won't for you, either. Heck, I'm *still* making changes and learning more along the way. Pick one action at a time and try it out in your routine. If it works, awesome! Now, move on to the next item. Baby steps, my healthy friend, baby steps.

We've focused on getting your bod to its highest levels of health, but—as I learned while mixing up my lemonade—your healthiest healthy also includes your mental, emotional, and social health, so let's tackle that in part two.

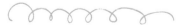

PART TWO

YOUR MIND

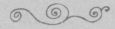

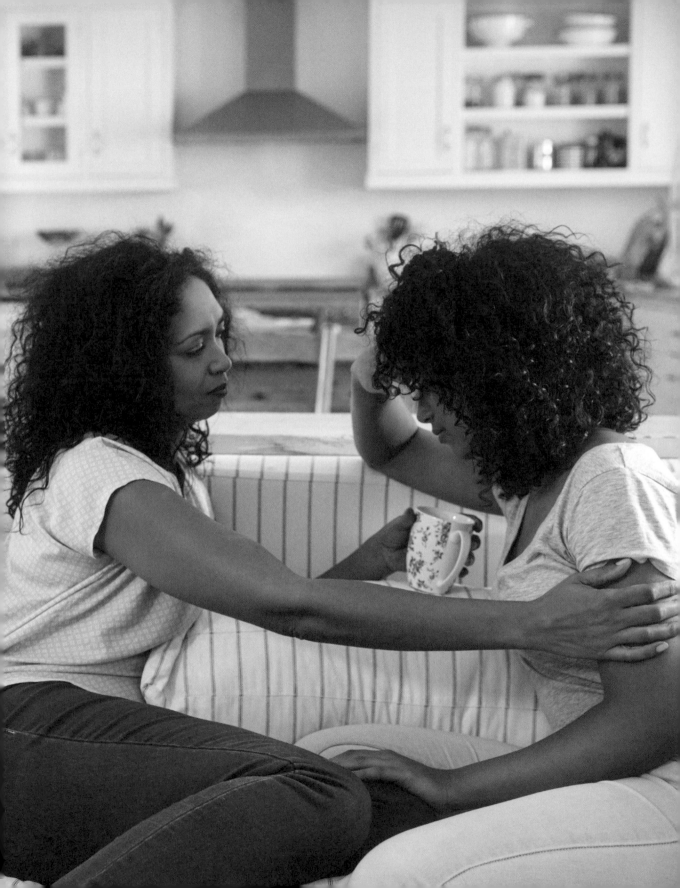

5

HANDLE YOUR HEALTH

After my diagnosis, my husband never missed one of my medical appointments. He stuck even closer to my side than in those first puppy-love days of dating. Postsurgery, when I couldn't lift my arms for weeks, he helped me change, washed my hair, and clipped my toenails. *Warning: gross detail ahead!* He even gave me an enema when all the medication impacted my bowels. Not exactly the back-door access that guys dream about. After nearly two decades together, Michael and I still don't pee in front of each other, so that, people, is true love!

More than anything, though, my cancer made us both realize the importance of communicating and showing our appreciation for each other—not just during a health crisis but also during the daily grind. My partner showed up. He was there. But I had to do my part by telling him exactly what I needed.

After a lot of discussion, we told our girls separately and slightly differently, essentially saying to both: "Mommy is

going to have surgery to take something out of her body that shouldn't be there, so she won't be able to get out of bed for a few weeks." We used the term "breast cancer" with our elder daughter, lest she hear it first from a kid at school.

After telling my family, I told select friends, most of whom totally supported me. Eventually, I wanted to go broader with my news. For me, it was easier to tell everyone all at once, rather than having it trickle out, group by group or person by person, which sounded more stressful. My mom and sister have always been incredibly important to me. Deciding to share my diagnosis outside the family proved especially scary because my father had died of colon cancer. My diagnosis brought to the surface painful feelings that would impact my family's lives, too. We talked about my decision, and I wouldn't have gone public without their blessing.

When deciding whether and how to "come out" about my cancer, the obvious dawned on me. Here I was, a healthy-

as-hell 40-year-old, walking around with a cancerous tumor. What if even *one* other woman had heard from a medical professional that her cancerous lump was "nothing"? What if my story could help her? That was enough. Shared stories have power, and Mama had a story to tell. *Roll cameras!*

I had made the decision, but seeing it in print in the tabloids meant no hiding from reality. My inner tiger wanted to fight off prying eyes and protect myself. After I got out of my sweatpants and traded my puffy eyes for a more determined look, I realized that I *needed* to talk to survivors to learn more: women who had survived this, families who had found a sweeter new normal. The more I spoke with them, the more I realized that either I could take control of the conversation about my cancer or I could let it become hot gossip. Before the article breaking my diagnosis to the world appeared, I made a list of close friends to call and called them. My people

needed to hear the news from me.

Now imagine seeing your most intimate health news splashed across the pages of *People* magazine, dissected inside *OK!*, *Star*, and *InTouch Weekly*, covered on *Entertainment Tonight* and *E! News*, and even discussed on *Good Morning America*.

"Samantha Harris Diagnosed with Breast Cancer; Will Undergo Double Mastectomy; May Need Chemo."

Yikes.

The small-town Minnesota girl in me worried that putting my story in a magazine or on the morning network news would fuel a backlash. Not the right kind of lemonade! Thankfully, survivors and others offered only unbridled support. The newsstand revelation hit like a shock wave. Calls, texts, and messages poured in from friends, acquaintances, and an incredible community of survivors. It was more overwhelming than my opening night on Broadway. That moment—the feeling of boundless love and support that could have filled 100 theaters—inspired me to launch GottaMakeLemonade.com (more on that in chapter 8). For total strangers to offer their help through something like this was a tremendous experience.

Even if it doesn't qualify as national news, everyone has her own version of a health coming-out story. Hearing the news about your body is just the beginning. You have to learn how to handle it, decide whether and how you want to share your journey with others, and then take care of yourself through that journey. So far, we've talked a lot about the tangibles in your healthiest healthy, but the intangibles—the mental and emotional strength and support that you build—are just as important as those morning runs and kale smoothies. Let's build 'em strong!

YOUR CRISIS SURVIVAL GUIDE

Hopefully you never end up in a situation where you have to say, "Mommy has cancer," or cry during sex the night before surgery (the last time I *felt* my husband feeling my boobs), or worry about how to tell your mom—not to mention the world—that you don't know whether you'll live a long or short life.

We all have to deal with some seriously sour situations at one point or another. That's the human experience. Whether it's a batch of passing bitterness or a life-changing diagnosis, handling a crisis can feel like an insurmountable challenge. But you got this! As with overhauling your pantry or your makeup drawer, take it one small step at a time.

First, you gotta take care of *yourself.* Here's how therapists Dr. Ellen Jacobs, LCSW, and Zachary Alti, LMSW, advise handling a health crisis on a personal level:

* **Take a deep breath.** In a holy $#!% moment, stay calm by reminding yourself that, no matter what's going on, you *can* get through it. Easier said than done, so start with one deep breath. That's right, just one breath. Then do it again.
* **Allow yourself to process.** Receiving devastating news can prove, well, devastating. Don't feel like you have to fight all your emotions and become a Zen robot in the first five minutes. Remind yourself that feeling angry, scared, and confused is normal and OK.
* **Ride the waves.** While you're riding the roller coaster, recognize that the waves of emotion are valid but also temporary. Every moment of fear and anxiety eventually will pass.
* **Follow up.** When you hear bad news, it can cause a physiological reaction— racing heart, light-headedness, nausea,

inability to focus. You might miss important information in those early moments of shock. Once you've had a chance to calm down and process, go back to your doctor to make sure you have all the info straight.

* **Call a friend.** But not just any friend. Contact someone who will offer calming, grounding support. This isn't the time for someone to freak out with you.

* **Speak up.** Don't be afraid to ask for what you need from your support network or to be direct about it. A lot of times, your nearest and dearest are waiting for clear instruction so they can be the best damn cheerleading squad, sappy-movie buddies, or bucket-list adventurers you need. Prioritize the logistical, emotional, existential, and financial support you need and be open about it.

* **Take breaks.** This is seriously a lot to handle! To stay strong, schedule self-care breaks and escape reality for a bit with a good book, a favorite TV show, or a yoga class to clear your mind.

* **Remember your badass moments.** Recall when you've faced challenges and made it through them. Even if this seems nothing like those past experiences, remembering moments of strength can help.

When I was first diagnosed, no one talked to me about the importance of self-care, but it's a *huge* part of getting through a health crisis and for finding your healthiest healthy. "Self-care is critical," says Dr. Jacobs. "It's the foundation of coping." In its simplest form, self-care means putting your needs first and soothing yourself. As a caregiver mama bear, I understand how hard putting your needs first can be. For me, that meant monthly—OK, weekly—massages at one of the cheapo Thai massage places near my house. Show your amazing self a little love with these easy self-care actions.

* **Lighten your load.** Slow down and make more time for what you truly enjoy. Everything else will still be there when you return.

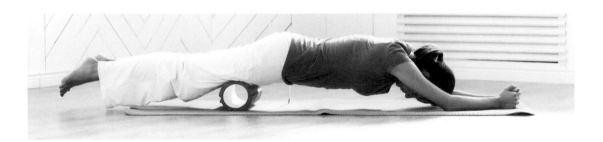

* **Get a massage.** Giving your bod some extra TLC is like giving yourself a giant hug.
* **Hit the gym.** When you're beyond frustrated about your situation, try kickboxing. Take a relaxing yoga class when you need some soothing.
* **Roll it out.** A regular foam rolling routine can make your body feel better—or try a yoga ball. No more kinks!
* **Meditate.** Quieting your mind can reduce your anxiety and make you feel better equipped to handle stress. (More on the benefits of getting your Om on in chapter 7.)

* **Commune with nature.** Studies show that spending time in nature helps silence nasty, self-critical thoughts, which can function as a key driver of mental illnesses, such as depression.[1] Yep, a simple walk in the woods can help clear your mental skies.

HEALTHY HACK

One study found that women with breast cancer could focus and take their minds off stressful subjects better after spending just two hours a week in nature. Even the C-monster is no match for Mama Nature![2]

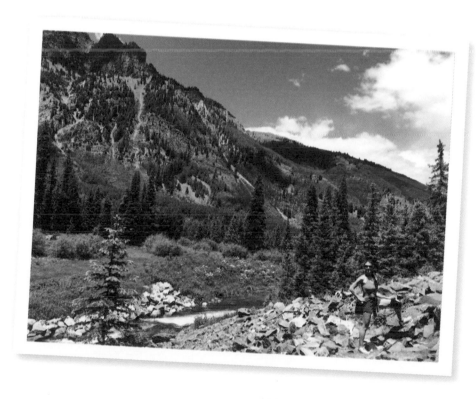

RELATIONSHIP SURVIVAL GUIDE

Really bad news can do a number on your personal psyche, but it also can sucker-punch your intimate relationships. We'll talk more about the importance of relationship maintenance and your support squad in the next chapter, but here's how to handle them immediately after a serious health bomb.

"One of the challenges in a relationship is that, when a difficult situation comes to a couple, both people are feeling pain at the same time," says Dr. Jacobs. "You're in so much distress that you can't always support each other as much as you'd like. That's when it can help to expand your network of support." Many times, that means reaching out to other members of your circle—sibling, bestie, workout partner—for additional help, but it also means *leaning into* your closest relationship. Trust me, your honey is handling enough right now—he or she doesn't need to play guessing games to figure out how to help.

How to Keep Caring

Relationships are a two-way street, so you need to say what you want or need, but you also need to show your love for your partner—even when you're fighting for your life. Here's how.[3]

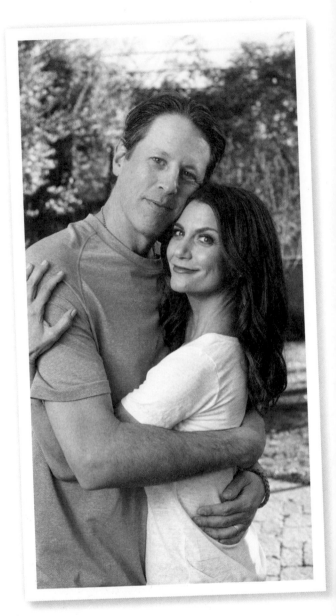

* Keep an appreciation journal by your bed. When you're feeling thankful for something your honey did, write about

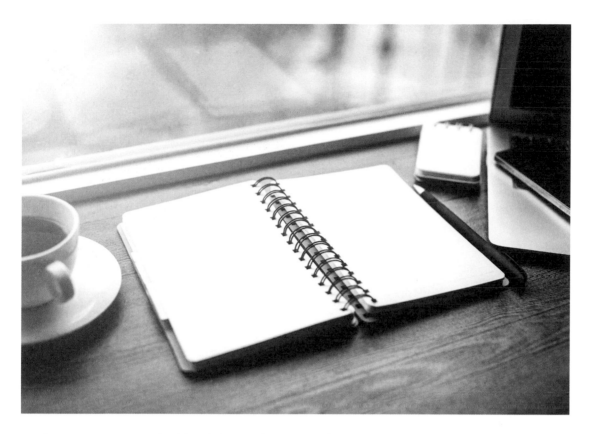

that on your partner's side of the book and vice versa.

* Take over your sweetie's least favorite chore.
* Pick up the latest issue of your partner's favorite magazine for him or her.
* Kiss before you part ways for the day— every single time.
* Be honest about sexpectations. If you're not feelin' it or if you want to but can't, don't leave your significant other in the dark. Just knowing that you want to get busy can help maintain a sense of connectedness.

* Sit with your honey during his or her favorite TV show even if you can't stand it. (*Big Brother*, again?! OK.)
* Send a random "love you, babe" text or, if you're feeling très romantique, write a love letter.
* Share a funny article you read to brighten up your lover's inbox.
* End your phone call more thoughtfully than an automatic "Love you, too."
* Ask your partner for a list of things that make him or her feel loved, then do one thing from that list when it's least expected.

CRISIS SURVIVAL FOR KIDS

Surviving crisis mode with your kids requires serious communication skills. It's one thing to talk to another adult about something as monumental as cancer . . . but your *kids*? To keep our family strong and healthy, I talked with pros—therapist friends and experts—who specialize in exactly this kind of situation.

According to them, the first rule is to be honest with kids. Withholding information or using euphemisms can cause anxiety and confusion later. "Younger children may use their imaginations to fill in the blanks, while older children may turn to the Internet, which could expose them to even more frightening scenarios than the one their family is facing," says Dr. Chrissy Salley, a pediatric psychologist who deals with sour scenarios every day. Words have meaning, so proper terminology has power!

Getting kids up to speed on any family crisis can prove tricky. How you navigate it largely depends on the crisis and the child's age. There's a big difference between what a three-year-old and a six-year-old can process. No matter how old the kid in question, keep two major points in mind:

1. Plan exactly what you're going to say before blurting out anything to a child, says Dr. Dana Crawford, a clinical psychologist who works with children. "My rule of thumb is

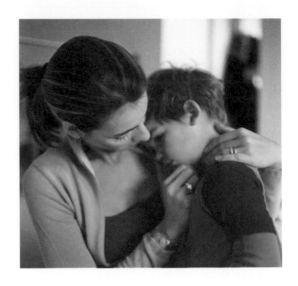

to share only as much as you are comfortable with."

2. Don't think of it as just one talk, says Dr. Salley. It's going to be an ongoing conversation.

HEALTHY HACK

If you're worried about how your child will handle the news, ask your doctor for recommendations for psychologists or social workers who specialize in helping families dealing with health crises. Also check out the Resources section at the end of this book for some great books on the subject.

Here, according to Dr. Salley, is how to break it down by age.

Age	What They Understand	How to Communicate
3–5 years old	Young children have excellent imaginations and often engage in magical thinking, which they sometimes use to fill in the blanks about subjects they don't understand. They can make unexpected assumptions or try to connect events or circumstances. They might even believe that they caused the illness.	Give basic information in simple but accurate terms. Avoid euphemisms ("boo-boo") even at this young age. Use the name of the diagnosis even if your little one can't pronounce it. It's important that children can differentiate this illness from their own experiences so that they don't worry that "being sick" or having a "boo-boo" means they will need the same level of medical attention that the parent is receiving. Explain that there's a plan (taking special medicine called chemotherapy, having surgery to remove a tumor) to help you get better.
6–12 years old	Children at this age want to know how the disease will affect their lives. Discuss what changes they can expect in the family, such as a grandparent or neighbor helping with transportation to and from school. By this age, children may have heard of the illness, so it's helpful to ask what they already know and to correct any misconceptions when talking about your situation.	Give specific information about the diagnosis and treatment. (Mom will have surgery next week to remove as much of the cancer as possible. She will be recovering at home for a few weeks, and then the doctors will see how she is doing. After recovery, she plans to have chemotherapy. We will talk more about chemotherapy as we have more information). Tell your children that you will keep them updated as you have more information or if something changes.
13–18 years old	With the Internet readily at hand, teens may stumble on information that can mislead or frighten them. You can't keep them from this, but you can direct them to reliable and accurate resources, such as cancer.org. When possible, sit with your teen and look at this information together.	Keep teens in the loop about the diagnosis, treatment plan, and updates over time. Older children, particularly older teens, may not want to talk about it so they don't have to think about what might happen. Take advantage of good opportunities to talk, but follow their lead and refrain from forcing them to talk about it.

These are the key points to make with kids of any age:

* Name the illness and give a simple definition of what it means.
* Emphasize that it has nothing to do with the child. Reinforce with younger kids that they didn't cause it and they can't catch it.
* Explain how you're going to treat the illness and the expected outcome of the treatment(s).
* Point out that it will change you. Prepare kids so they know what's going on if you start losing your hair or don't have the energy to play with them.
* Tell them that any major health issue means changes to the family. Specify how the situation will change their routines and what you'll do as a family to stay in sync.
* Underscore that they will still receive proper care during this time. Daddy may be on lunch duty. Gramma may come to stay for a while.
* Stress that your door is always open. Let kiddos know that they can talk about it whenever they need to. Knowing that you're OK with talking about it will make the future seem less scary for them.

One of the best ways to help kids cope is to make sure the news isn't all bad. According to the experts, making simple, positive routines part of your new normal can help you and the kids make some lemonade together. "Small rituals can be huge," says Dr. Crawford. "It's not so much the amount of time you spend but that the parent is clearly labeling the activity 'our special time together' or 'our special thing.'" I told my girls we could start taking food from the kitchen containment zone for after-school "picnics" in our bedroom while I was confined to bed. Fun new projects, such as making bracelets, braiding hair crowns, and designing doll dresses also became part of our special time together. Lemonade everywhere!

GOING PUBLIC

Once the shock has passed and you've navigated those early moments of crisis, you have to decide how to talk about those lemons. That likely starts with the people closest to you—spouse and/or kids—which we've covered. But what about your boss? Friends? Workout buddies?

"It's a very personal thing," says Dr. Jacobs. "There are no rules about how people deal with illness. Everyone has an absolute right to share or not share." In other words, this is *your* story. Deciding whether, when, and how you'll talk about your health with anyone else is totally up to you and, when done right, can help you cope. No TV broadcast required, I promise.

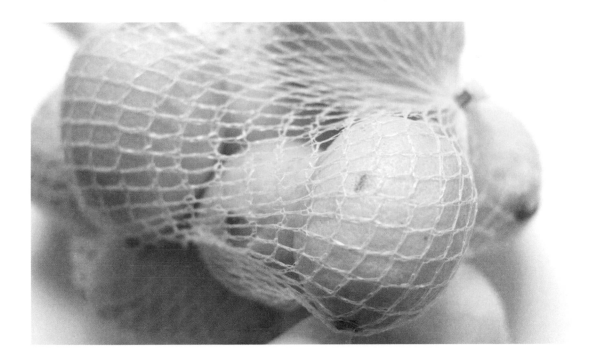

Let the Lemons Out of the Bag

You don't have to shout your diagnosis from the rooftops or share it all over social media the second you leave the doctor's office. It's totally OK to sit with it for a few days or weeks before sharing it with others. Then start small with your must-tells. See how it feels with your closest crew and go from there. Remember, you need to put *your* needs first, and it's OK to preface a conversation with that point, says Dr. Jacobs. As with everything else in this book, take small steps first. Dr. Jacobs suggests asking yourself the following questions to help you decide whom to tell and how.

* **What's your reason for sharing?** Do you want to talk about it? Do you want the person to support you? Do you need to explain why you're suddenly sluggish or dropping weight faster than you should be?

* **Will it be more stressful not to share?** If keeping mum will drive you mad, let it out.

* **What will the person do with this information?** Some people can't help using information to their advantage. Your cancer diagnosis is yours to share and no one else's. If you tell someone, will the person keep your news confidential?

* **Has the person been supportive in the past?** If someone has a history of flaking, ditching you in times of need, or amplifying your anxiety, think twice about telling.
* **How does the person handle stress?** Even with the best intentions, some friends can't help but flip over bad news. Will this person provide a source of support or just lose it?

Don't forget that going public can impact other people in your life. Discuss it with them first. Whether your story appears on your social media newsfeed or the evening news, sharing can be powerful and have a meaningful ripple effect, bigger than belting a high C! An amazing community is out there for you if and when you need it.

advice—right away. Yeah, not always helpful. Anxiety is contagious, and you have enough on your plate without having to assuage the doomsday worries of those around you. "You need to communicate with people what you need," says Dr. Jacobs. "Don't be afraid to be direct." Which means that sometimes you gotta say thanks but no thanks.

It's OK to say:

* I want to share this news, but I'm not ready to talk about the details. I'll let you know when I am.
* I'm working with a bunch of awesome experts, so hearing opinions from everyone else is making me feel anxious. Let's talk about something else.
* This conversation isn't helping me right now. Why don't we talk another time.

HEALTHY HACK

You've decided whom to tell and how (face-to-face, phone, etc.), but what if you're not sure what to say? Try practicing what you'll say with someone who already knows the news or write a list of bullet points or a script for yourself.

THE FEEDBACK LOOP

Now that your lemons are out of the bag, prepare for others to offer unsolicited

HEALTHY HACK

Having a formal conversation about what you need and what you don't can feel draining after a while. Establish a code word or phrase with family or friends that lets them know when you need to change the subject without having a long, serious talk about it. Try: "We should grab a lemonade" or "Gee, I love Broadway" or "Unicorns!"—or your favorite trigger word.

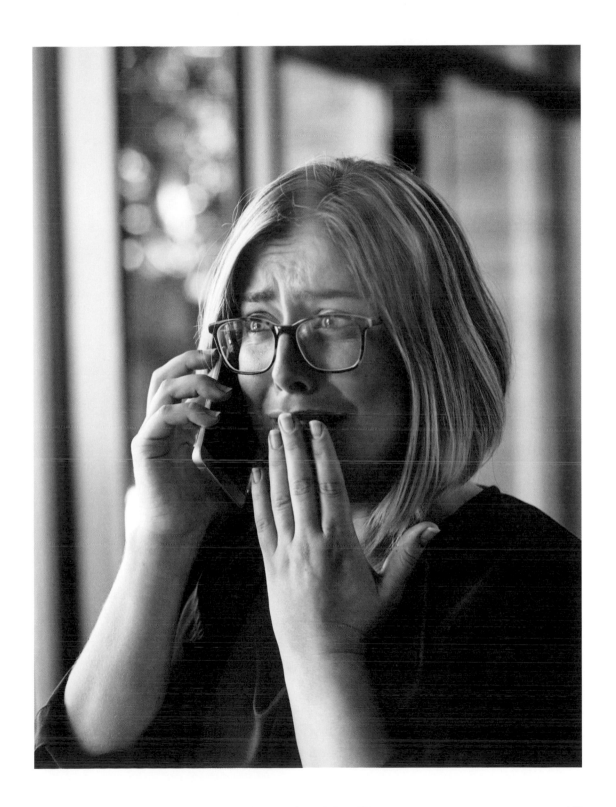

SURVIVAL GUIDE FOR LOVED ONES

This section is primarily for the partner or other loved one of the patient, so just for this section "you" means the patient's partner or loved one, rather than the patient.

Being the partner, sibling, best friend, or any member of the support squad for someone going through a cancer crisis or other scary health diagnosis is a hell all its own. "We think of pain and illness as something that happens to us as individuals, and that's just not true," says Matt Lundquist, LCSW, a therapist in New York City. "We experience them collectively with those around us." Here's how my incredibly supportive hubby, Michael, handled my health hell:

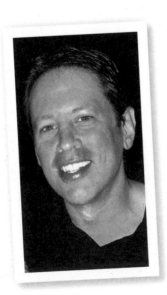

When I got the news of Samantha's diagnosis, it was the first moment the thought, *I might outlive my wife*, had ever occurred to me. How would I live without her? How would I know how to raise girls? After the confusion and panic had passed, I wanted to be strong for her and help our family in every way possible—whether that was helping her get in and out of bed or bringing some levity into the cancer chaos.

My role started with just being there physically at every doctor's appointment and mentally by talking through every option, every hope, and every fear together. Then it meant supporting her decision to have the mastectomy, even when I didn't agree initially. (Her surgeon originally recommended a less invasive lumpectomy plus radiation, but strong-willed Samantha made up her mind to have the mastectomy, and I'm glad she did.) It meant going over lists of pros and cons together and finally recognizing that the peace of mind she has now, because of the mastectomy, is way better than the what-ifs that would have driven her crazy.

Samantha is the ultimate caregiver; she often puts our needs ahead of her own. I honestly underestimated what it would be like to take on that role for our family. It scared me to have to take care of my strong-as-hell wife. It got to me. Meanwhile, feeling like a "burden" was hard for her. (This from the woman who shocked all the nurses by insisting that she go for a walk just hours after her surgery—I mean, *who does that?*) I am so proud to watch her handle her health with such grit and hold our family to a higher standard.

On the other side of it, our partnership definitely has grown stronger. We realized on another level just how lucky we are to have each other and our girls but also how lucky we are to have our health. It's important to pay that forward. Because finding our healthiest healthy is so important to her, it's important to me, too.

That's my man!—and you, the caregiver, are probably having some of the same thoughts and feelings. If you don't know where to start or what to do, the first thing to say is nothing at all. Just listen, then acknowledge what you heard and respond with empathy. Here are some simple but effective responses.

* I'm so sorry you're going through this.
* I can't imagine how difficult this must be.
* I'm so proud that you're facing this challenge head-on.
* It's going to be a difficult journey, and I'm with you every step of the way.

You should offer your support, of course, but that looks different from person to person. Sending a bunch of WebMD articles to a friend who writes for a health magazine probably isn't helpful.

How to Offer Kick-Ass Support
Hearing the C word, whether that's cancer or another major crisis, can feel like a diagnosis for you as well as your loved one.[4] If your main squeeze or another loved one is fielding a major health lemon, these expert-backed tips will help you rock your spot on the support squad in her time of need.[5]

Don't Ask, Tell

Sometimes a person in crisis doesn't know what help she needs, let alone how to direct you. Asking how you can help can feel overwhelming. Instead, say what you're going to *do*.

SAY "I'm going to bring you dinner every Tuesday and Thursday. Do you want whole wheat pasta primavera or veggie burgers this week?"

Gift Generously

After my surgery, a friend and fellow breast cancer survivor brought me her special body pillows to help me sleep, positioned on my back throughout the months while my front bits recovered. That gesture meant the world to me.

GIVE something you know your loved one needs or will enjoy. Think beyond flowers and food. If you're not sure, ask the doctor or nursing team about favorite recovery gifts that patients find super useful.

Pick Up the Slack

The last thing a cancer patient wants to worry about is the grocery shopping, laundry, or dry cleaning. To keep errands and chores from adding stress, pick up the slack like a merry little house elf.

RUN errands and do chores on preset days. Have your loved one write down anything that comes to mind during the week and take care of everything on the list on those days.

Think of Yourself

Channel the golden rule and use your imagination. If you were in her shoes, what help would you want? Focus on the practical: eating healthy food every day, showering, and so on.

LIST everything you would want your own support squad to do for you. Share that with your loved one and let her order the services that *she* wants. A little à la carte menu!

In case you haven't noticed already, relationships are a big deal. They represent an essential step in reaching your healthiest healthy. Now that you can handle the news and you've shared it with the people you want to know about it, you need to ditch the toxic people in your life and forge even stronger bonds with the good ones. You so got this!

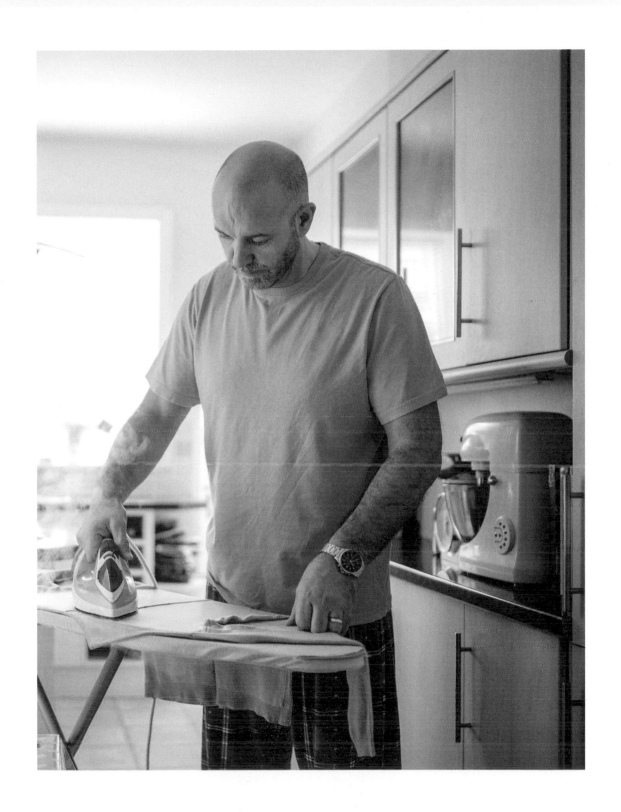

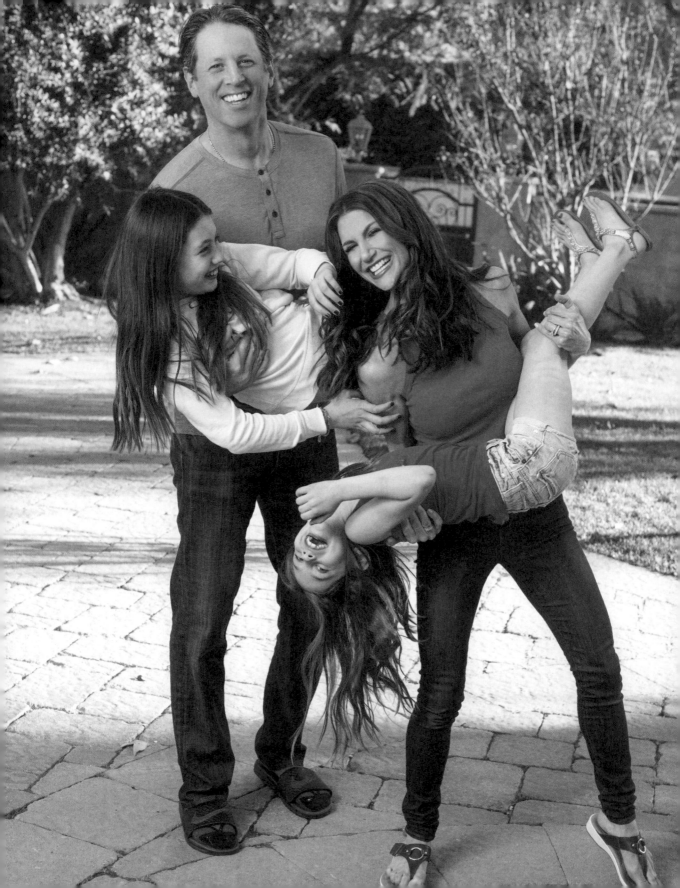

6

GET REAL WITH RELATIONSHIPS

My husband and I try to keep our libidos limber. My V-card stayed with me until well into my 20s, but once I got into the swing of things, I was a boob girl in the bedroom. Before my surgeries, he and I had a bon voyage celebration for my ta-tas. Modern medicine can recreate pretty natural looking ones, but docs can't yet recreate the feeling from fondling. Losing that sensation left me feeling robbed and vulnerable. Imagine if one of your favorite spots suddenly went numb! But like many women with a cancer diagnosis, my libido slipped into granny panties, footy pajamas, and then a coma. These days, sex—specifically matching my bod's responses to my desires—forms a big part of my healthiest healthy.

When I came home, bloody and bruised from both of my surgeries, my husband and mini nurses held my hands the whole way up the stairs, helped me change into my jammies, and, in little Hilly's case, even helped empty my surgical drains with all the fascination of a future doctor (ew, but fingers

crossed). For months, my health hijacked their lives just as much as it did mine.

My support squad—mother, sister, stepdad, step-sis, in-laws, and friends—came out in full force in my time of need. They jumped into the ring with a pair of pink boxing gloves: meal deliveries, nurse-maiding, helpful reading material, and endless conversations on the phone or at the end of my bed when I needed to chat. All that bed rest created a forced meditation retreat for my normally career-focused, pedal-to-the-metal brain. For the first time in years, I had a chance to watch the shows that sparkled as the crowning jewels in my career. Having to stay in bed gave me perspective: My family motivates my life. Being my healthiest, best self for them and supporting them so they can be their healthiest, happiest selves—those are my goals.

During those early days, when my body wasn't ready for sex, making sure my partner knew how much I still desired him mattered to me. Some days truly challenged me, but I wanted him to know that he wasn't losing the woman in me. That in turn reminded me that I wasn't any less of a woman without my breasts. It helped me feel empowered, invincible, like I could belt out a few bars of Helen Reddy's "I Am Woman." Cancer or no cancer, I still wanted my sex life.

Nothing creates anticipation like weeks of bruised and bandaged boobs—*so* sexy. When we finally got it on, it took some adjustment. We both had to find a new normal. In Michael's case, that meant understanding that fondling my new breasts wasn't going to hurt me. But that didn't stop us from *being* together. Just as in the early days of our relationship, we took small steps to rediscover our sweetest sex life.

That wasn't the only physical change we experienced as a couple. Let me explain: My hubby was never a runner. When we first met, he still had his basketball-player physique from his college athlete days, but, as with so many marriages, gym time fell by the wayside. My loving invitations (*cough*, nagging) to get his butt in gear with me at the gym weren't about wanting to rub my hands all over a muscular man (well, not primarily anyway). My dad died when I was 22 years old, and I want my daughters to have *two p*arents to walk them down the aisle. Urging him to exercise with me was about ensuring that he stuck around for the long haul, not about six-pack abs. (But, hey,

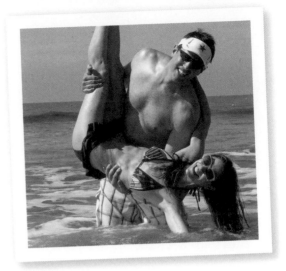

if his workouts come with a hotter bod in bed, who am I to object, right?)

None of my prodding worked until he read a book by one of his buddies about training with a Navy SEAL. He devoured it in one day, and the next day, while I was lying bleary-eyed and bewildered in bed, he jumped up at 5 a.m., amped to hit the treadmill. *What the—?* Something about the book got under his skin, resuscitating his discipline. He started running regularly, dropped 30 pounds in three months, joined me for morning smoothies, and even bet a coworker he could run 750 miles by the end of the year. That's more than half a marathon every week! He finally uncovered his healthiest healthy. (See how powerful books can be? Hint, hint!)

But his journey was bigger than just improving his body. Six months into his new routine, he wanted to show our girls that, when you set your mind to it, you can accomplish amazing things. So he picked a date, started training, and a few months later he ran 50 miles on a 1-mile track to prove that he could do it. That's right, a couple of years into my new postcancer normal, my hubby ran a solo 50-mile ultra-marathon in one day. While earning plenty of bragging rights, he made his newfound health a family affair. We supported him while he trained, and he shared the rewards with us by turning his challenge into Family Race Day, which allowed our girls to set and crush their own goals and gave me the opportunity to finish my longest run ever: 18 miles, baby!

The point of that story is that health challenges can feel isolating. Being part of a family—the one you were born into, the one you created, the one you assembled for yourself—means being part of a team. Your support squad holds your hand, figuratively and literally sometimes, cheering as you cross the finish line on the track or in the hospital. Ultimately, you have to endure and overcome early morning runs or scary surgeries, but it's a *lot* easier when you have a supportive community around you—whether that's two people or 2 million. Deepening these loving relationships in your life and pruning when necessary both sweeten your lemonade and function as a key ingredient in your healthiest healthy.

It's not just about sweating together, though. As my kids grow older, the cancer conversation in our household has grown up, too, evolving into a more detailed discussion about family health history. My girls know now that cancer took my dad's life early, but they also understand that my cancer was different. My elder daughter heard me talking about it on the phone when she was nine years old. "Wait! You mean you could have *died*?" she said. Watching her grasp that fact for the first time was heart-wrenching, but honest, age-appropriate conversations lead to great questions and answers.

Just as the most important relationships in your life help you find your healthiest healthy, here's how to share your newfound healthy goodness with the people you love.

SWEETER SEX LIFE

Sex can play a huge role in the emotional recovery process, because feeling desired matters. "Having a healthy sex life means having a normal sexual response when you want to, becoming aroused when stimulated, and being able to have pain-free sex with orgasm," says Dr. Lauren Streicher, medical director of the Northwestern Medicine Center for Sexual Medicine and Menopause, who specializes in treating sexual health issues postcancer.

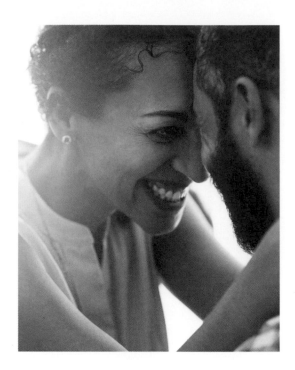

HEALTHY HACK

If you don't have a lot of libido or if you're experiencing sexual dysfunction as a result of dealing with a health issue, there's hope, says Dr. Streicher. "The number one thing to get across to women is that there are solutions. If someone has told you otherwise, they're wrong." Ask your gyno to refer you to an MD who specializes in sexual medicine.

If your libido's in good shape, you can benefit from the pleasures of sex. It's a little like a case of chicken and egg, but studies suggest that regular sex helps insulate blood pressure levels from stress, boost neuron production, and lower anxiety. It's even been associated with better cognitive function in older adults.[1] Regular frisky time also might help you feel healthier. In a study of more than 3,000 adults, researchers found a positive association with self-reported health. In other words, people who had more nookie felt healthier.[2] Hot damn!

Another reason to get it on regularly? "There is a lot of truth to the idea of 'Use it or lose it,'" says Dr. Streicher. "We know that women who are having vaginal intercourse on a regular basis are less likely to experience vaginal dryness, tightness, and pain, which a lot of women experience as they get older." If you're experiencing issues in that department, or especially if you're dealing with sex in the context of cancer, talk to your doctor. Regular hanky-panky won't prevent all below-the-belt issues, and you might need more help, Dr. Streicher adds.

Keeping intimacy on point years into a marriage is hard, but keeping it alive in the face of cancer or another serious health diagnosis is a whole new ballgame. Sometimes sex really is like going to the gym. Some days you may have to give yourself a little extra push to get there, but you'll feel better once you do. Aww, yeah!

Remember, you are your own sex goddess, and some days (or months) you just won't want to get it on. That's OK! Stressing out about not having enough sex isn't exactly going to help your health now, is it?

Your body doesn't define who you are. Even when you can't control it, you can do something about how you feel and express desire. "A lot of people think sex is the same as intimacy. It's not," says Dr. Streicher. In other words, even if intercourse is off the, um, table, that doesn't mean intimacy is. "There are lots of ways to be sexual and lots of ways to be intimate." Here, from the sexperts themselves, is how you can continue stoking the fires of love, no matter what your physical situation.

* **Get close.** Sex, which is only one form of intimacy, is often off-limits for a variety of reasons in any relationship. Physical affection and closeness are equally powerful. Holding hands, cuddling together, or sleeping naked are all great ways to build intimacy. —Dr. Franklin Porter

* **Talk dirty.** If you're feeling sexual or missing your sexual connection, talk about it. If you're in the mood, talk about what you want to do when you're well again. Share what you miss most about your physical bond. —Rebecca Hendrix, LMFT

* **Expand the menu.** It can be a wake-up call when you aren't able to have the same relationship with your body. Develop a new sex menu that has different ingredients, where intercourse isn't the main course. Realize you can make love with more than just your genitalia and start making love with your hands, mouth, and brain.—Dr. Ian Kerner

* **Be together.** Spend time together doing things you love. Think of activities you used to do when you first met and see what's possible now. If you can't go see the Rolling Stones, watch one of their concert films together. If you both enjoy games, play cards or your favorite board game to have some normal experiences together. With a cancer diagnosis, you can't avoid many heavy, intense moments. Create moments of normalcy with some joy or laughter to offset the heaviness. —Rebecca Hendrix, LMFT

HEALTHY HACK

Even without a major health crisis, the daily grind gets to us all. To prevent your partnership from turning tepid, make showing the love a priority. Award points to whoever initiates sexy times after a long day, and trade them in for disliked chores, first pick of a film, or 10-minute backrubs. Win-win!

SEVEN STEPS FOR A BETTER SEX LIFE

Whether you're reeling from a diagnosis or dealing with a desire-killing daily routine, you can benefit from a little extra sweetness in your sex life. Here are seven steps to help you get there.

1. **Appreciate each other.** A sweet sex life starts with a sweet relationship, which means remembering—and communicating!—everything you love about your honey on a regular basis. "Acknowledge or appreciate your partner for one thing every day," Rebecca Hendrix, LMFT, recommends.

2. **Stretch when not in sync.** Your sex drive won't always align perfectly with your partner's, and no matter how much your honey-pie is into you, getting frisky every time your inner sex kitten purrs might not happen. That's perfectly OK, says Hendrix. "Sometimes you will have to stretch, and sometimes your partner will," she says. "Sometimes you will have to agree it's just not a good time to have sex without taking it personally."

3. **Have sex talks.** No, not the dirty kind. "Sex becomes the elephant in the room only when you aren't having it," says Hendrix. "Before the elephant settles in for a stay, discuss its arrival." This isn't about playing the blame game, though. It's about checking in with genuine curiosity. Does your partner think something is off, too? What might be behind it? How can you *both* turn this around?

4. **Turn yourself on.** The one person most responsible for your sexual self is you. "We are sexual beings, but everyday life can leave us out of touch with our sexuality," says Hendrix. Take care of your sexual self with solo time when needed. "Most of us are too tired or overloaded mentally to switch our minds and bodies into being sexually open. If this is you, ask yourself what you need to become sexually open. It may be a bath, meditating, certain music, or aromatherapy." Or maybe just a great vibrator!

5. **Turn your partner on.** Leaving a little to the imagination can help reignite a spark. (For example: Avoid spousal enemas at all costs!) Reinvigorate your relationship by leaving sexy notes, pictures, or hints about a fantasy for your partner to find in private. Sexy texts in the middle of the day can set the tone for some lovin' later on.

6. **Switch it up.** There's nothing wrong with a routine that works, but even the most surefire moves can grow stale. "There's a place for familiarity and a place for novelty in the bedroom," says Dr. Ian Kerner, a certified sex therapist and author of *She Comes First.* "You have to be conscious of those two separate poles." If you usually get it on at night, dabble in some morning glory. If you're always in the bedroom, give the couch a spin. (Just be sure the kids are away for a sleepover!)

7. **Don't take it too seriously.** Have some freakin' fun! "Laughter can be an automatic mood changer," says Hendrix.

FAMILY-FRIENDLY FOOD

Your Healthiest Healthy involves showing all your relationships more love, from sexytimes to the family life that follows. As a woman, you know why making all these changes is so worth it. The kale smoothies don't taste as good as a chocolate milk shake, but ultimately they're *way* more satisfying, energizing, and health-ifying. As adults, we get that. A five-year-old, however, has a much looser grasp on why salad is good and soda isn't.

Early habits die hard, though, and they can wreck our long-term health in the process. Studies show that childhood obesity leads to all kinds of health issues throughout the life span, including adulthood obesity and increased risk of type 2 diabetes, cardiovascular disease, and several cancers.[3] Even eating too much animal protein around puberty can affect the future breast cancer outcome for your kids, according to *The China Study.*[4] Just as for us mamas, knowledge and understanding help kids make decisions that lead them to form healthy lifelong habits.

HEALTHY HACK

Treat "fat" as a bad word—not the nutrient in food but in any conversation about anyone's body. Your healthiest healthy isn't about body image. You want to teach your little ones from the get-go that the choices they make are about having their healthiest—not cutest—bodies. Period. It's about what their little bods can *do* for them. Eat veggies to make you strong. Gobble beans to run faster. Stay away from sneaky sugars to fend off diseases.

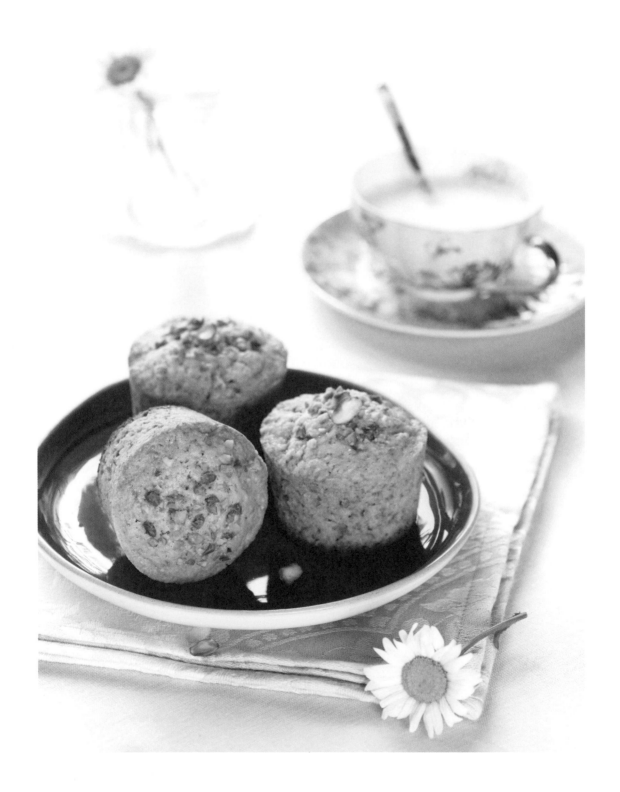

YOUR HEALTHIEST HEALTHY

FAMILY-FRIENDLY RECIPES

Kiddos love getting into everything in the kitchen, and these recipes can help channel that curious energy. The prep is easy for little hands to assist, and they'll delight in the results.

Shrek Muffins

YIELD **12 muffins**   PREP TIME **35 minutes**   COOK TIME **15 minutes**   TOTAL TIME **50 minutes**

Getting kids to eat anything green can make for a real struggle, so get sneaky with fun names they can't resist.

* 1 tablespoon chia seeds
* 2 tablespoons coconut oil, plus more for greasing
* ½ cup unsweetened organic applesauce
* 4 large organic eggs
* 2 teaspoons vanilla extract
* 2 cups organic spinach, fresh
* 1–1½ bananas, ripe
* ¼ cup organic pure maple syrup
* 1¼ cups almond flour
* ¼ cup coconut flour
* 1 teaspoon baking powder
* ½ teaspoon salt
* ½ cup crushed pistachios (optional)

1. Soak the chia seeds in 1½ tablespoons cold or room-temperature water for 10 minutes or more.

2. Preheat oven to 350°F and grease a muffin pan with some coconut oil.

3. In a high-powered countertop blender, blend the first 8 ingredients on high until smooth.

4. Add the remaining ingredients and puree for another 1 or 2 minutes.

5. Fill the muffin cups ¾ full, top with pistachios if using, and bake for 15 minutes.

6. Let cool and, to absorb excess moisture, place paper towels beneath and in between layers of muffins before sealing and storing in the refrigerator.

Breakfast Ice Cream

YIELD **12 ounces**   PREP TIME **10 minutes**

Nothing beats ice cream for breakfast, but it's *healthy* "ice cream." You can sub 4 to 6 ounces of cashew milk for the yogurt and mix and match your favorite frozen organic fruits. The more ice you add, the more this turns into a frozen treat. Extra credit if you add ½ tablespoon chia seeds and keep things organic!

* 1 banana, peeled and frozen
* 1–1½ cups frozen organic strawberries
* 6 ounces plain nonfat Greek yogurt
* 2 cups ice or more
* 1 splash unsweetened vanilla-flavored almond or cashew milk (if using yogurt)

In a high-powered countertop blender, blend all ingredients on high until smooth. Be careful not to overblend or your ice cream will become a smoothie!

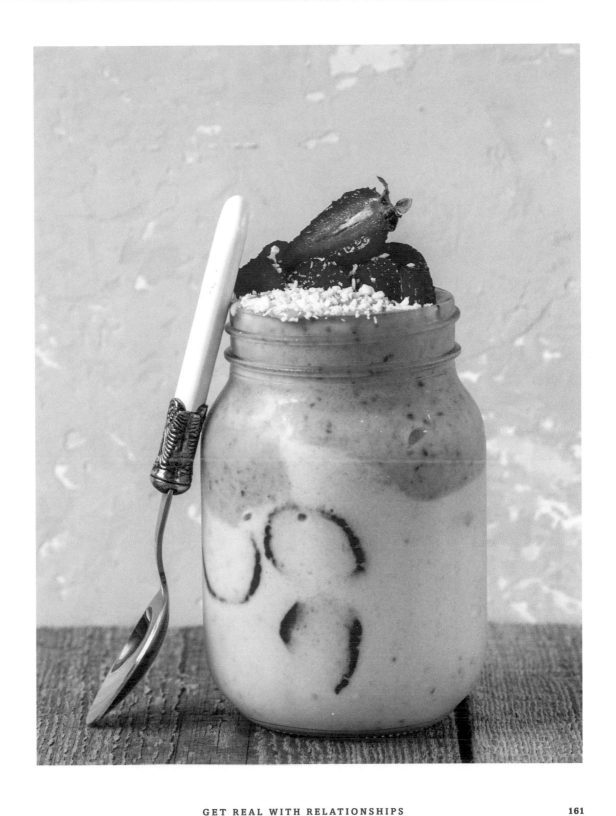

Power Pasta Primavera

YIELD **4 servings**   PREP TIME **30 minutes**   COOK TIME **15 minutes**   TOTAL TIME **45 minutes**

If chicken appears at nearly all your dinners, use this yummy recipe to wean your family off poultry and onto some plant-based protein. Feel free to substitute red lentil, green lentil, or black bean pasta and your favorite veggies.

* 1 bunch asparagus
* Himalayan salt
* 1 large head organic broccoli or 2 small heads
* 1 (12-ounce) jar roasted red bell peppers
* 1 or 2 cloves garlic
* 1 teaspoon extra virgin olive oil
* 1 (25-ounce) jar organic marinara or vodka sauce
* 16 ounces chickpea rotini
* 4 tablespoons freshly grated Parmesan cheese

1. Trim ends of asparagus and cut the spears into 1-inch pieces.
2. Drizzle the spears with extra virgin olive oil, sprinkle them with salt, and broil them for about 10 minutes, keeping a careful eye on them so they don't burn.
3. Cut broccoli into bite-size pieces and steam them in a pot with 2 inches of boiling water. Keep covered but vented, until bright green, about 5 to 8 minutes.
4. Boil a large pot of water for the pasta.
5. Chop the roasted red bell peppers.
6. In a large pan, sauté the garlic on medium heat in the extra virgin olive oil for 2 minutes or until tender and fragrant.
7. Add the sauce to the pan and stir in the red peppers. Cook on low while making the pasta.
8. Cook the pasta according to the package instructions.
9. When the asparagus and broccoli finish cooking, add them to the sauce and simmer for 2 to 3 minutes.
10. Toss everything together and top with Parmesan cheese.

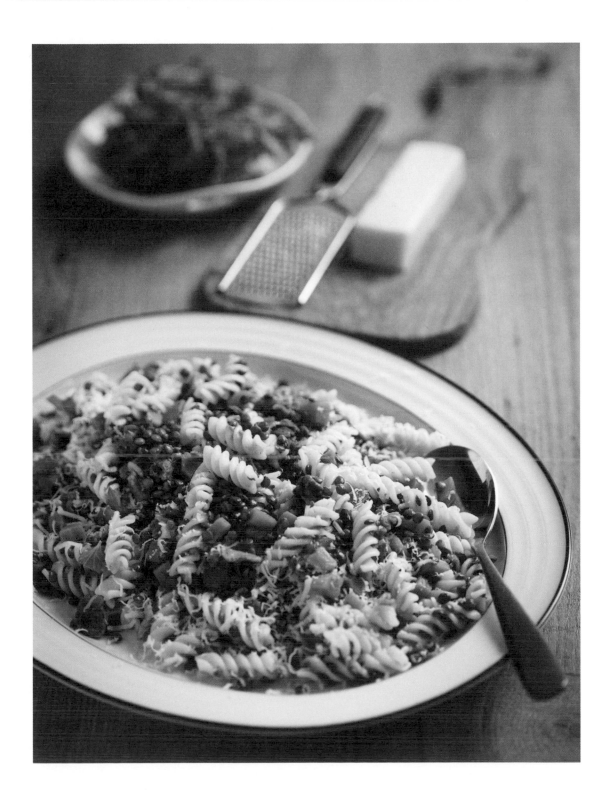

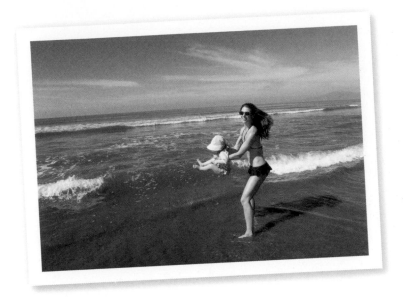

FAMILY-FRIENDLY FITNESS

Just like food choices, it's important to model positive body practices for the whole fam. Joining the school dance team or gymnastics squad isn't about staying skinny, it's about building body confidence. When my daughters were really little, they were part of my fitness routine. (Imagine doing squats or stair-climbing with a 20-pound baby strapped to your back.) Now that they're older, we turn fitness into family fun.

These activities will help foster a genuine love of exercise, rather than making the gym a drill-sergeant mandate. They also can help keep your bod in tip-top shape when playdates and carpools hijack your HIIT classes. Plus, a little family fitness doubles as quality time with the kiddos.

* **Play tag.** Nothing builds a love of cardio like running for your life from whoever is "it."
* **Jump rope.** Brush off your double-Dutch skills for this throwback activity. Jumping rope for 15 minutes burns about 150 calories.
* **Go old school.** Throw it back even further with other oldies but goodies, such as a wheelbarrow race or hopscotch.
* **Hit the playground.** Turn your local playground into a family-friendly fitness park. Challenge your kids to contests on the monkey bars to build upper body strength. Work your hamstrings by pumping to reach (safe) new heights on the swings. Get some cardio by racing up the ladder to the slide.

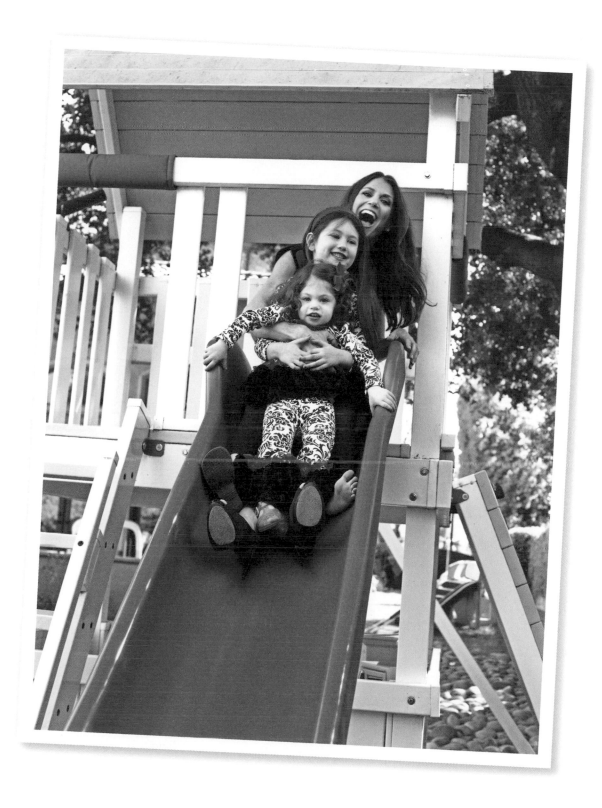

* **Take a ride.** Start a postdinner tradition of going for a bike ride and get your kids used to the idea of sticking to a daily routine.
* **Make it a destination.** A weekend walk or low-intensity hike to a favorite breakfast spot offers a reward for the effort, which can help motivate the kids.
* **Hit the pool.** Swimming and pool games help kids burn off all that extra energy, and they love channeling their inner mermaid or shark. Turn all that splashing into a solid workout. Challenge each other to handstand and somersault contests or swim tag.

KEEP IT KID-FRIENDLY

One of the best things about finding your healthiest healthy is that, in discovering healthier nontoxic products, you can pass on tons of healthy goodness to your little ones without worry. My journey also helped me find the best care team for my kiddos and talk to them about grown-up health realities in a way they can handle.

Beauty Products

All the nontoxic products we discussed in chapter 3 are kid-friendly, so no extra research needed. Phew! If you wouldn't use something on your kids, you shouldn't be using it on your own body, either. Some of my favorite products for me are designed *for* kids. When the little ones want to play "makeup salon," you can have a fit over the mess instead of the toxins.

Pint-Sized Doc Squad

You know the importance of building the best team for yourself, so do exactly that for your minis. Many of the same rules apply, but for kids you want to deal with pediatric specialists whenever you can, says Dr. Darria Long Gillespie, so look for a pediatric dentist and, if your kiddo falls off the monkey bars, as mine did, a pediatric orthopedist.

Keep the Conversation Going

Short of having a crystal ball (if only), genetic test results can give you the clearest possible understanding of what lies in your kids' future. If your own test results reveal worrisome markers, such as a hereditary cancer gene, talk to your family doctor about how to use that information to monitor your kids' health as they age and when it might be appropriate to have them tested.

If you have a family history of a particular illness, being open about that with kids can help them understand the importance of the health foods section of the grocery store and regular trips to the doctor. The strategies for communicating with kids from chapter 5 don't stop applying once a crisis has passed. Use the chart on page 141 as a tool to keep talking!

SUPPORT SQUAD

In my experience, you will encounter two kinds of friends in times of crisis, whether that's something as fleeting as a traumatic experience with a bikini wax or as serious as a cancer diagnosis. I call them the Positive Pollys and the Negative Nellys.

"When we're surrounded by people who want to show us love and support, that's going to impact how we experience challenges," says Matt Lundquist, LCSW, a therapist in New York City. Having these Positive Polly reinforcements makes any battle easier. Research suggests that having a solid social group can encourage you to be more active, and people with strong social relationships live longer, according to a meta-analysis of 148 studies.[5]

But your squad also can release shrapnel. You know these friends: the ones who make every conversation about them, knock down your moments of triumph, breed anxiety, or just plain suck at making plans and keeping them. The Negative Nellys zap your energy and take more than they give. Not ingredients in your healthiest healthy. "We've all tolerated these negative

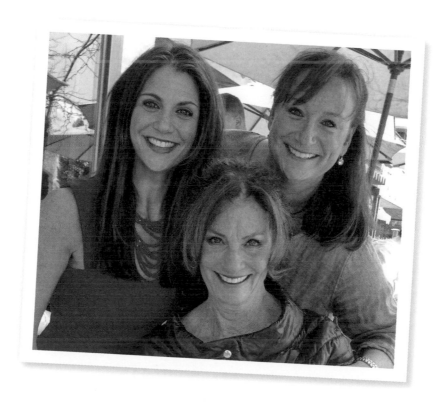

behaviors, but the stakes are higher after a crisis," says Lundquist.

Negative vibes are literally contagious. It's called Emotional Contagion Theory.[6] We humans are wired to mimic the physical and social cues from the people around us. It's how we've learned evolutionarily to avoid embarrassment and shame and relate to our social circles. So science says it really does matter whom you surround yourself with. Ditch those toxic relationships, just as you ditched those toxic tampons.

"This is a mega upside of a crisis— it's a great opportunity to clean house," Lundquist says. That can be tricky, though, because friends don't come with ingredients lists and EWG warnings (again, if only). People also react to trauma in unexpected ways. But doing due diligence on your crew to see who's not measuring up can help you say sayonara to the Negative Nellys and knock out that negativity with a one-two punch! Pink boxing gloves optional.

THE NEGATIVITY QUIZ

If you're feeling overwhelmed and can't figure out who's helping or just getting in the way, think about and honestly answer these six questions.

1. **Who's not showing up for you?**
   Dealing with life's lemons is hard (duh). Good friends don't run for the hills. They show up with a juicer. "Listen to what people are telling you in both word and deed," says Lundquist. Which friends are getting on a plane, bringing you dinner, or regularly calling to check in? The ones who aren't are worth a closer look.

2. **Who's changing the subject?**
   "People might change the subject or conveniently need to go when that topic comes up," Lundquist says. Consider that emotional ghosting in your time of need.

3. **Who's making it about themselves?**
   "When you're going through a crisis, you're in a place where what you need is kind of about you," says Lundquist. It's important to take breaks from that and talk about other things, but a friend who makes your crisis about what's scary or stressful for *her*—or seems jealous of the attention you're getting—has gotta go, *stat*.

4. **Who's trying to control things?**
   In an effort to be helpful, a gal pal might take over the situation by bombarding your inbox with research on treatments, making appointments you didn't ask for, or constantly questioning your decisions. Not kosher. Care and control are two

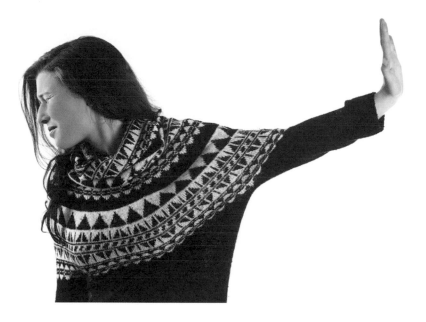

different behaviors, and you have room for only one in your support squad.

5. **Who's being too positive?** Sometimes the Negative Nellys can masquerade as overly Positive Pollys. If someone tries to cut you off with cheery statements any time you start to talk about anything scary, it's "a polite way of saying 'I'm not available to have this hard conversation with you,'" according to Lundquist. What's going on may be tricky or scary, but you still need to be able to talk about the sour stuff.

6. **Who's not meeting you in the middle?** With certain friendships, you make all the effort—always meeting them on their side of town, scheduling playdates, calling to catch up. Their *mishigas* may be detracting from an egalitarian friendship. Is that relationship really adding anything meaningful to your life? Focus only on the relationships that do.

At first, it felt selfish to cut a conversation short or to turn down an invitation. But one of the ways that having cancer helps clarify your life is that even lovely people sometimes aren't right for your support squad. We have more important things to worry about, my healthy friend.

HOW TO DROP A TOXIC FRIENDSHIP

Breaking up with a friend can cause more anxiety than ditching a lover. "If someone isn't showing up for you, it's important to recognize that," says Lundquist. "Stop acting like you're not seeing what you're seeing." Ultimately, you want to be honest and straightforward to dump the toxic relationships in your life with as little stress as possible.

Be Direct

Be gentle, but don't worry about being delicate. "This is a rip-the-bandage-off kind of conversation," says Lundquist. "When we try to be subtle, we end up with the worst of both worlds where we're not really articulating the message and then we don't feel satisfied."

Put your issues out there by saying: "Hey, this thing really bothers me, and I've noticed it's kind of a pattern." You might be able to clear up a misunderstanding or deliver a wake-up call.

Manage Your Expectations

Don't get your hopes up about a movie-screen happy ending. "People who have the audacity to be mediocre friends or to drop you in a crisis also tend to do a pretty poor job of looking in the mirror when their bad behavior is called out," Lundquist says. "It's really unlikely that that person is going to get it and apologize." More likely, they'll just get defensive. Prepare accordingly.

Brace for Backlash

Stay calm and make sure you've got those boxing gloves in self-protection mode. "Going into the conversation, think about what would be most helpful for you in terms of ending the relationship and walking away with less negativity in your life. Put your needs first," says Lundquist. "The number one priority is making sure you don't get slimed."

Finding Community

Beyond your support squad, larger communities offer another sweet spot for your healthiest healthy. After I shared my story publicly, I attended a Look Good, Feel Better workshop, a program developed by the American Cancer Society and the Personal Care Products Council. This workshop addresses the aesthetic issues that often accompany a cancer diagnosis and have an emotional impact (learning to put on a wig or draw on eyebrows). The woman next to me said, "I'm so glad I could talk to you about my cancer because no one in my family knows. . . . I haven't told anyone."

That sentence still breaks my heart. We all need community and support.

At my lowest—lying in recovery after surgery—my husband took my hand and said, "Babe, sometimes you just gotta make lemonade." He was right. Thinking about it for the next few days made us both realize that making lemonade wasn't just a cliché. Having cancer sucks. So does losing a loved one. So does getting fired. So does going through a rough breakup. Every day, life dishes up lemons. So let's gather together and turn those lemons into something better.

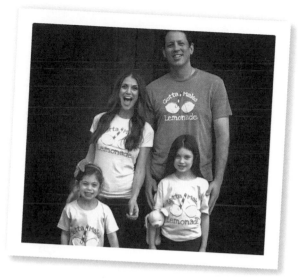

That's why Michael and I created Gotta Make Lemonade (GottaMakeLemonade.com). It's an online community where people share stories of finding positivity in the face of adversity, gather support, and take away kick-ass gems of goodness that help them get to their healthiest state of social, mental, and physical health.

This isn't just some lovey-dovey mumbo jumbo, either. The research on the benefits of communities is solid. A 2016 study found that the more groups you're a part of, including family and friends, the happier you feel.[7] (See, girls' nights totally are good for you!) Our communities give us the strength and support to survive life's challenges.

My support squad and my greater communities helped me turn cancer into a journey to my healthiest healthy, which is pretty awesome—if I do say so myself!

Gotta Make Lemonade got me there. (Keep an eye out for some stellar inspiration in chapter 8, where I'll share some of my favorite GML stories.)

＊ ＊ ＊

By now, you've packed a pretty amazing toolkit for reaching your own healthiest healthy: best eating habits, a badass body plan, a field guide for a toxin-free life, an all-star team of health experts, a crisis survival guide, and strategies for assembling the best team of cheerleaders. Good job!

But to keep movin' and groovin', you also need the tools to build a positive and resilient mindset. So grab your Positive Pollys and let's talk about the power of positivity when it comes to your health!

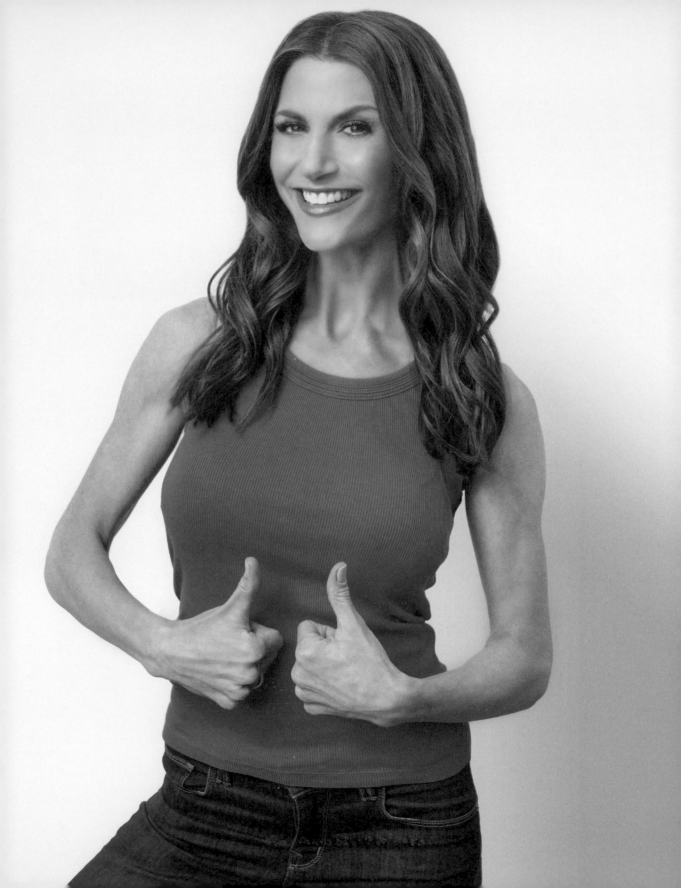

7

PRACTICE POSITIVITY

When faced with a roadblock, throwing a smile has always been my best punch. At age 11, I asked my parents for an agent to help me navigate Minnesota's oh-so-glamorous commercial acting and print modeling scene. The red carpets were a long way off, so my glass-half-full attitude developed really fast. Every time I didn't get a part, the little optimist in my brain shouted, *Can't knock me down! I'm gonna get the next one!* Positivity was shooting out of my twinkle toes as if I were a Disney princess.

In seventh grade, a bunch of older girls read a list of lies about me in front of the entire lunchroom. It was like something from *Mean Girls*. The world is full of idiots and jerks. You can't control what they say, but you can control how you react. That realization, which came years later, gave me power.

Moving to La La Land dropped another sucker punch on my positivity, especially while I was struggle-juggling three jobs for years. But when success came my way in Tinseltown, my positivity muscles got their most challenging workout ever. Stepping into the public eye—whether on a social media feed or national TV—means that people are going to offer unsolicited opinions. No, Internet stranger, I don't care that you think I have no neck or that you think I sound like a man on *Dancing with the Stars*, thankyouverymuch. That's life.

Then cancer happened.

Of course, even my inner Positive Polly couldn't avoid life's regular onslaught of sadness, butterflies, and fears, but the C-monster ravaged me with anxiety like I'd never experienced. Suddenly cancer was controlling me. Replacing my natural perkiness, a constant adrenaline panic made me want to hyperventilate, throw up, or have a tabloid-worthy meltdown. Not good. That wasn't a sustainable way to deal with my diagnosis or my life. Long-term sulking just isn't my style. It was time to channel my starry-eyed, 11-year-old self to get back on the path to positivity.

As you've gathered, I'm a gym geek. Getting my sweat on helps me feel accomplished, focused, and present. In some of my darker moments, a good workout helped sub for a long cry on the phone with my big sis. Otherwise, one of my favorite ways to pursue that kind of body-to-brain positivity is through yoga. I probably first tried it because Madonna said that's how she got her freakishly toned arms or something. (Seriously, have you seen her arms? #Goals.) On the path to my healthiest healthy, my borderline burning-up relationship with yoga took a holiday. My nonstop life needed a ray of light. Yoga forced me to slow down and show more love to my *mental* muscles.

Believe me, it wasn't all rainbows and sunshine the whole way. Plenty of days left me feeling totally knocked down and wanting to curl into a ball and ugly-cry, *Real Housewives*–style. We all have those days, and that's OK. Seriously. It's important to deal with how you're feeling, whether you're ready to shimmy into your booty jeans and conquer the world or you're dangling an inch away from crawling into bed and admitting defeat. By choosing the positive path, even on rough days, I could acknowledge my fears and not have to deal with them alone. Having cancer helped teach me this incredibly valuable lesson: You always can choose to meet your anxieties and fears with a positive attitude.

That kind of positivity is one of the most potent ingredients in your healthiest healthy. But let's be real. Practicing positivity is easier said than done. If Disney princess optimism doesn't come naturally to you, that's OK. You can train your brain just as you trained your taste buds in chapter 1 or your muscle motivation in chapter 2. Let's see how.

PRACTICE MAKES POSITIVE

Practicing positivity starts with recognizing your reality—bitter bits included. It's OK to put on rose-colored glasses, but not blinders. The reality of my new cancer normal started with accepting the truth.

Samantha, you have cancer.
OK, got it. Now, what's positive in this situation?

Well, we caught it super early.
Good, keep listing.

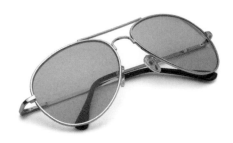

I'm in a much better place financially than many women who receive this diagnosis every day.

That's a blessing worth counting. What else?

I have the most amazing support system and my otherwise good health will make recovery faster.

See, not so bad.

To stop the negativity spiral, you need to throw a wrench in that anxiety engine, says Dr. Danielle Shelov, a clinical psychologist. "If we can slow ourselves down and recognize our anxiety, we often can stop the negative spiral before it begins." Start small. Go for a walk, do some meditative yoga, or use self-talk (as I did above) to change your thought patterns. "The brain can learn and be retrained to loop in a less reactive way," Dr. Shelov says.

Those rose-colored glasses don't always go on easily, though. Getting them in place takes small steps. Practicing positivity means choosing to change your thought patterns. Just as with a new gym routine, it starts with little changes and ends with big gains. When you feel the shadow of negativity creeping closer:

* Stay present. Tackle your concerns when you need to address them but don't spend your whole day worrying about something looming in the future.
* Focus on what you can control.

* Remind yourself of the good things you have going.
* Question the reasoning behind your worries.

Also remember that cultivating a positive mindset doesn't mean slapping a smile on everything, which can prove counterproductive. "Letting someone share their negative and often worrisome thoughts and feelings can accomplish an important goal," says Laurie Sloane, LCSW, a psychotherapist. Negative thoughts and feelings are OK as long as you deal with them in a positive way. In other words, you can't hide life's lemons and still make lemonade to drink.

This isn't just Pollyanna pseudoscience, either. Yours truly, a peace-and-love Cali girl, respects cold, hard science, and the research on the power of positivity is vast. Psychology professor and researcher Dr. Barbara Fredrickson found that experiencing positive emotions, such as love, joy, and contentment, affects you in many ways.

* **Positivity changes your brain.** After starting a positive meditation practice (more on the benefits of that later), participants reported increased mindfulness, sense of purpose in life, social support, and overall life satisfaction.[1]

* **Positivity changes your body.**
  Participants also reported physical improvements, including decreased symptoms of illness and depression.[2] How 'bout them apples?

These two upsides of a sunny disposition comprise the Broaden and Build Theory. Positive vibes spring you into action and open your mind, which promotes the discovery of new things, places, and people. That, in turn, increases your physical, mental, and social resources.[3] How cool is that? Happyville does exist!

HEALTHY HACK

To help you stay positive, research suggests that you use social media wisely. Studies have drawn a link between logging on and decreased happiness both in the moment and over time.[4] Further studies have shown that it's all about *how* you use social media.[5] As a tool for comparison, social media sabotages positive vibes, but it can be healthy for your headspace as a way to stay connected with others. Follow inspiring accounts and limit interaction with people who stoke your green-eyed monster.

BODY POSITIVITY

One of the cardio coaches at my gym likes to say, "You can choose to be strong, or you can choose to be weak. You can choose to be happy, or you can choose to be miserable. What do you choose?" That's right, some of my most inspirational pick-me-ups come from my home away from home. Sorry not sorry.

We tend to think of a positive outlook as all mental, but a surprising amount of science points to using our bodies to score positivity points. As we saw in chapter 2, exercise delivers almost as many brain boosts as body benefits, and research shows that getting your body moving can help prevent and treat clinical depression and anxiety effectively.[6]

For years, yoga sounded like a total snoozefest to me. If you think its slow and methodical movements seem boring or that it isn't a "real" workout, the Energizer Bunny in me totally gets it. But hang on.

First, a regular practice does have major body benefits. How do you think I got my Chaturanga arms? (Thanks, Madge!) Yoga boosts muscle strength, endurance, and cardio-respiratory fitness and encourages more mindful eating—a healthiest healthy cocktail of goodness![7] Research also shows that yoga helps you ditch negative thoughts and reach a more positive state.[8]

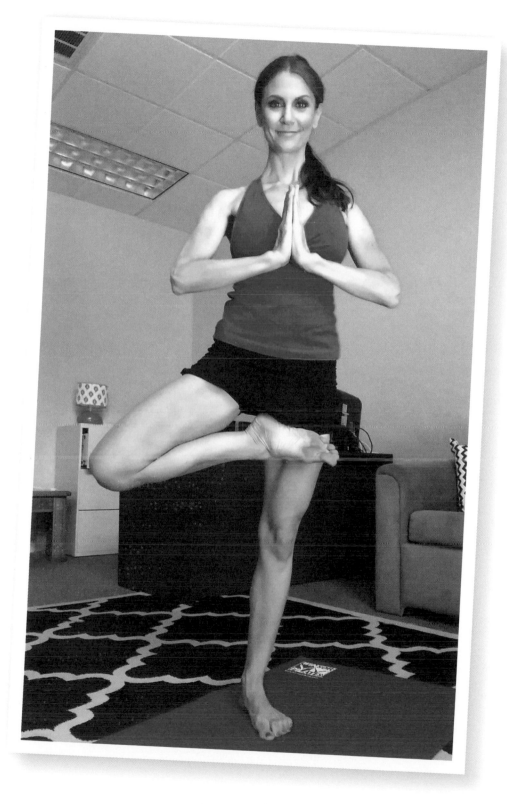

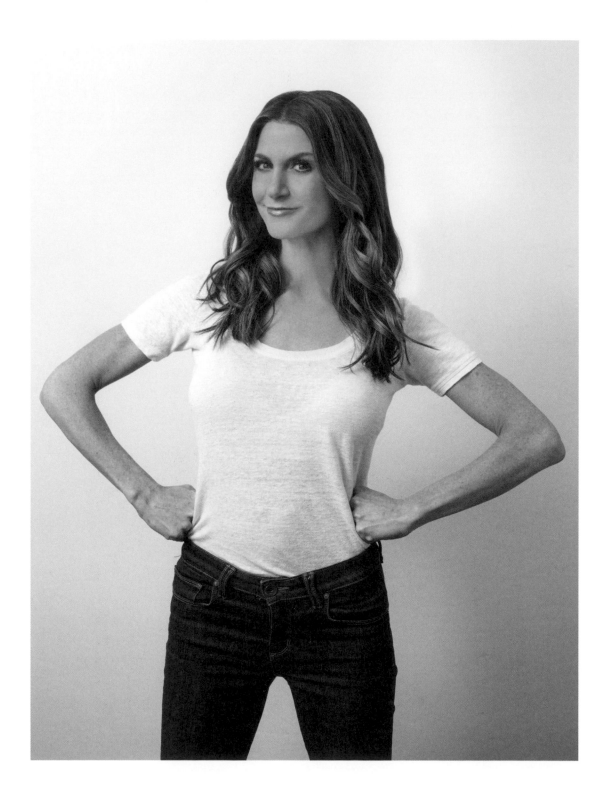

If you can't get to a full-on class or want to start small, begin with a couple of simple poses. Check out some of my favorite easy yoga routines on YourHealthiestHealthy.com or in the plethora of apps available, including Down Dog. (See the Resources section on page 201.)

The Power of Posing

Some studies indicate that you can harness the power of positivity with even subtler changes to your body by adjusting your posture. The theory, called Power Posing, comes from Harvard Business School professor Dr. Amy Cuddy.[9] The premise is simple: Put your body in a more powerful position—shoulders back, head held high, feet hip-width apart, hands on hips—and you'll *feel* more powerful and positive.

Cuddy's research suggests that doing your best Wonder Woman impersonation might change your brain chemistry. Her study found that adopting an assertive, expansive posture can increase your levels of testosterone and reduce your levels of cortisol (the stress hormone). Other scientists haven't been able to replicate her results, so the hard science is still controversial.[10] But test subjects reported *feeling* more powerful, so pull back those shoulders and fake it till you make it![11]

Beware, though: Power Posing theoretically works both ways. Slouching, crossing your arms, or shrinking into a corner can conjure up feelings of depression and sap your strong mindset, so watch your body language, especially when you need an extra jolt of confidence—like when you're walking into your doc's office with a long list of health questions.

THERE'S NO PLACE LIKE OM

Your bod needs periods of recovery to stay healthy and become healthier, and so does your brain. "Why do we not take care of our minds the way we do our bodies?" Dr. Shelov asks. Great freakin' question! When you work your biceps and your triceps, you can see your hard work in the mirror, but working your gray matter often results in a case of out of sight, out of mind, according to Dr. Shelov. Neglecting your mental fitness by not taking regular brain breaks can screw with your relationships—ever snap at a loved one for no reason?—and leave you in an unhealthy stress cycle.

So say hell-Om to a meditation routine. Its benefits rock. Studies show that it can:

* increase happiness[12]
* abolish anxiety[13]
* quash stress and boost self-love[14]
* promote better emotional control[15]
* mitigate pain[16]
* improve immune function[17]
* zap chronic inflammation[18]

My never-stop energy level means that meditation and I have a complicated relationship, so it's an ongoing struggle to make it a daily practice for me. But, hey, as I keep saying, finding your healthiest healthy involves a constantly evolving set of goals. This is one of mine. Making meditation part of your day-to-day wellness routine, even on a small scale, will help, and you can find a lot of steps between stress tornado and Zen master. Life pulls us in 5 million different directions all at once—kids, career, home, hobbies, passion projects, and more—so it's important to find simple strategies that work. Try these.

* **Go for two.** No matter how busy you are, you can carve two measly minutes from your day. Commit to two minutes of meditation time every day for one week . . . then another week. Before you know it, you'll be on your way to a positive practice. C'mon, I believe in you!

* **Set a time or a trigger.** To make sure you do it daily, set an alert on your phone for a convenient time, such as riding the train to work or sitting in the carpool line waiting to pick up your kids. My trigger is pulling into my parking spot. Not a bad way to start a workday!

* **Make a meditation zone.** Getting your Om on is a lot easier when you have a quiet place to concentrate. Turn a corner of your bedroom into an Om zone with a comfy pillow to sit on and a (nontoxic) beeswax candle. "Carving out a quiet space can be as simple as a few throw pillows on a rug, some greenery, a beautiful candle, and natural light," says interior designer and author Nate Berkus. "No clutter is key, and no devices. Our homes should tell our story and support us in taking care of ourselves. That means actively creating areas in our space that let us do that. Your home should 100 percent reflect how you want to live and feel."

* **Be present.** If meditating feels too hippy-dippy for you, sit quietly and take stock of your surroundings. How does the rug beneath you feel? What does the room smell like? How many seconds does it take to exhale a full breath?

* **Take it to go.** If all that stillness still isn't working for you, take your meditation on the move. Go for a walk. Rather than thinking about the office or dinner, focus on your breath, how your body feels, and the details of your surroundings. Pay attention to the sound of birds chirping or the warmth of the sun on your (SPF-protected) face.

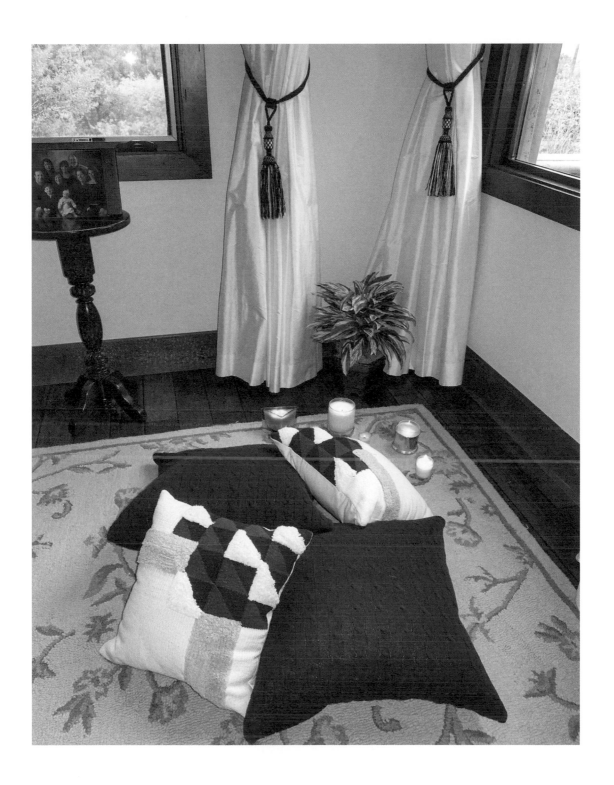

PRACTICE POSITIVITY

Take mini-meditation moments—just a deep breath to slow down and center yourself when you're feeling particularly frazzled.

Mantra Meditation

Getting into the meditation groove can prove tough, so Kathryn Budig, an internationally renowned teacher and Instagram yogi, offers this easy, guided method. For beginners, she recommends mantra and japa meditation.

Mantra meditation is super easy and starts with picking a mantra—something simple but personal. What do you need to affirm or reinforce about yourself? What reassures you? Mine, for example, evokes my inner Positive Polly: "I am healthy and happy. I am fit and strong." To meditate, think or say the first statement as you inhale and the second statement as you exhale. Repeat for the duration of your session.

Japa meditation is pretty similar, except that you use a necklace of mala beads and touch a bead each time you repeat your mantra. "These are both action-driven, which tend to give people a sense of

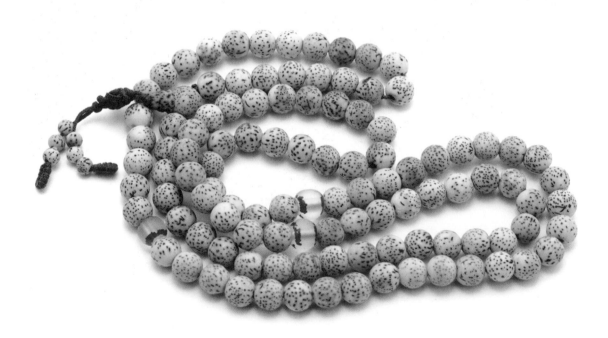

purpose, instead of feeling lost with sitting and trying to still their minds," Budig says. "In the morning, I use the mantra, 'I am energized. I am focused.' In the evening, 'I am calm. I am focused.' I'll do this for one to five minutes to get my head straight or to help slow it down."

Take a Brain Break

If sitting cross-legged, chanting, and trying to find your center makes your eyes roll, you can score a healthy mental boost by taking regular brain breaks, which help ensure that your mind gets the same level of rest and care as the rest of your body. These breaks tap into your gray matter's default mode network (DMN), a fancy term for the place your mind goes when your thoughts wander. Your DMN is damn important for lots of aspects of well-being, including intelligence, creativity, and memory formation.[19] Here's how you can build mental breaks into your day and engage your DMN.

* **Switch off.** I get it. We're all so flipping busy, but switching off doesn't have to mean sitting still in a silent room. When tackling the mindless repetitive items on your to-do list—dishes, laundry, chopping veggies—let your mind wander. Healthy zoning out *and* the chores get done—double yay!

* **Unplug.** This may come as a shock, but the world won't end if you turn off your phone. Instead of checking emails, scrolling through social media, or listening to a podcast, let your brain go off-leash for a little bit. Unpacking and processing your day will put you in a more positive mental state.

* **Take your lunch.** Even if it's just for the 15 minutes it takes to walk to and from your favorite salad place, leave your phone at your desk and let your thoughts roam free. Bonus points for eating it outside (if you can) and getting some fresh air.

* **Get some green.** Studies show that just being in a forest environment can lower cortisol levels, blood pressure, and switch your brain into chill mode.[20] If you're in a concrete jungle, make time to sit or walk in a nearby park or green space.

Practicing positivity the same way you practice the perfect lunge will give you a leg up on achieving better health and happiness. Go, you! Now get ready to arm yourself with strategies for building resiliency throughout your journey— along with some Disney princess–level inspiration to keep you movin' and motivated!

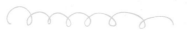

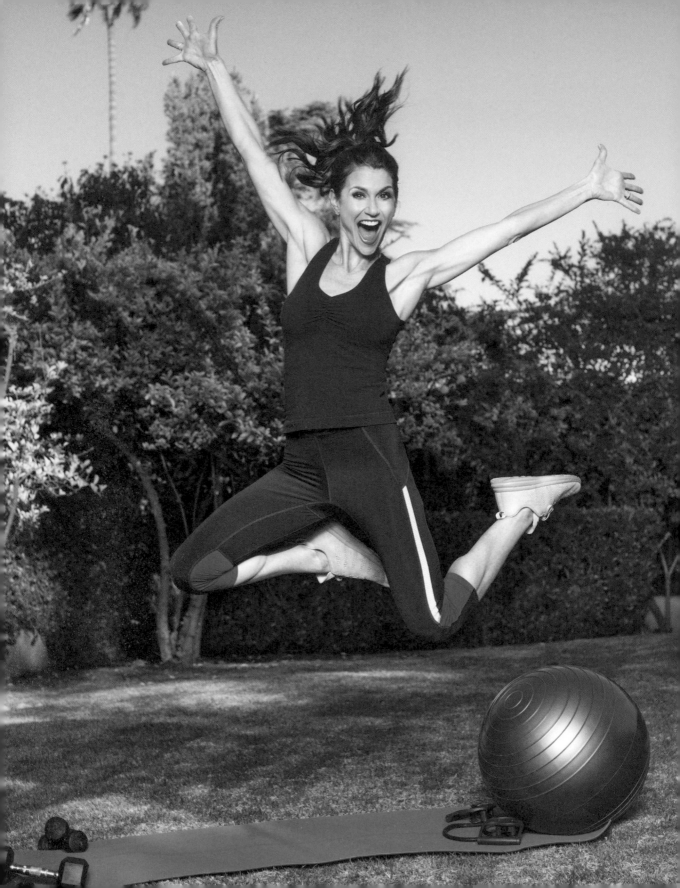

8

REV YOUR
RESILIENCY

ife has taught me that it's critically important to gather a supportive team around you, but in the end *you* are your own best health cheerleader, advocate, and defender. This journey—facing the scariest moment of my life, navigating a labyrinth of overwhelming health information, and ultimately finding my healthiest, happiest, most energized self—in many ways has become the best thing I've ever experienced. It has made me so much stronger as a survivor.

That's not because I learned to like kale or even because I chose to be fierce when facing seriously bad news. According to the experts, our ability not just to survive but to *thrive* after a setback is a psychological phenomenon. It's called Benefit Finding Theory. It's about "deriving positive growth from adversity."[1] Sounds a lot like the journey to your healthiest healthy, no? It's easier and more effective when you have solid social resources, such as your healthiest healthy relationships and communities, so let's hear it again for those support squads![2]

The challenges you face in life don't have to make you a victim. Instead, seize the reins and make a change toward better health and a happier, more energized life. You are not your adversity. You are not a statistic. Health challenges happen, but you can respond with a high kick to the face of those monsters and make them work for you. "Resiliency is the critical piece of what makes people survive and thrive," says Dr. Shelov. "It's hard to build, but the more resilient you are, the more you realize *you* have an impact on your own life." In other words, resiliency is the key to a survivor's mindset.

Your healthiest healthy is all about focusing on what you can control. Make the best choices possible and take small steps that are better for your body, brain, and well-being whenever you can. That's what I want this book to give you: an expert-backed road map out of the labyrinth, the tools to help you on your journey, the skills to stay the course, and a knockout sense of empowerment that you *can* do this! You *can* be your own best health advocate, and you *can* reach your healthiest healthy.

GET YOUR GOALS

We've set a lot of goals so far. (Shoutout to you, my healthy friend—woot woot!) Making sure they're the *right* goals is the first step to staying on track and developing the best long-term relationship with your health. Remember when we talked about intrinsic versus extrinsic motivation?—(page 53). That's what the experts call setting process goals versus outcome goals. "Process goals are based on action that we can control, while outcome goals are based on results," says Dr. Jonathan Fader. Not only are outcome goals not as healthy, but they can have major limitations. Here's how the difference looks in the real world.

Outcome goal: "I want to lose two dress sizes before my high school reunion."

Process goal: "I want to work out four days a week between now and my high school reunion so I feel sexy and confident in my new dress."

See the difference? Wanting to drop a dress size or two may be the universal struggle that unites women everywhere, but it's rooted in wrongheaded thinking. What if, after weeks of working out, you don't lose any weight, but you do lower your blood pressure, increase your endurance, and build some killer muscle tone? Does that mean all your hard work was for nothing? Will you feel like a failure on the big night? Like hell you will, mamacita! Those benchmarks mean success, and you should celebrate them with a couple of spins on the dance floor. (Bonus points for doing the Running Man, my favorite '80s dance move.)

Process goals have a leg up on outcome goals for two reasons: They concentrate on what you can control rather than an outcome that's out of your hands, and they focus on the effort you put into every mile—not just crossing the finish line—so you can feel good about them no matter what. Ground every step you take toward your healthiest healthy in this way of thinking. It's healthier for your mind and body, and it's more effective. Research proves it![3]

YOUR HEALTHIEST GOALS

A 2017 study found that writing down your goals makes you more likely to crush them.[4] So grab a pen! It's time to put your commitment to achieving your healthiest healthy on paper.

Why Do You Want to Reach Your Healthiest Healthy?
This is your primary intrinsic motivator, the reason you're here, the desire that's kept you reading every last nugget of health goodness so far.

_____

_____

_____

_____

Process Goals
List three more reasons, plus your process goals.

Physical Health Goals

(e.g., schedule recommended screenings, replace one meat meal per week with plant protein, focus on what you can achieve the next time you hit the gym)

_____

_____

_____

_____

_____

_____

Mental Health Goals

(e.g., meditate for two minutes every day)

Social Health Goals

(e.g., tell your partner or best friend something you appreciate about him or her each day)

Write Down the Small Steps You'll Take (or Already Have!) to Get There.

(e.g., checking the screening chart on page 119 or setting a meditation trigger)

GOTTA MAKE LEMONADE

No matter what kind of challenge you're facing—a health diagnosis, a struggle to better your brain and your body, a frustrating stagnation with your job or relationships—we all need a little inspiration from time to time. The stories shared by the amazing community on Gotta Make Lemonade often inspire me to keep going (even when I just want to cry), and they've helped inspire many other people, too. Here are some of my favorite recipes for lemonade (edited for content and clarity) to inspire you when the struggle feels all too real. These and many more are waiting for you to read on GottaMakeLemonade. com. While you're there, share your story with us, too!

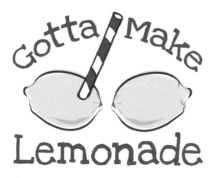

From Stage-3 Breast Cancer to Living a Fuller, Adventure-Filled Life

Being diagnosed with stage-3 breast cancer at age 34, amid an economic recession that forced my small business to close, was my lemon. Choosing to live a life full of accomplishments and goals that I knock out year after year is my lemonade.

Faced with the postcancer construction of a new normal to replace the life that was in ruins because of it, I made a list: 40 things to accomplish by my 40th birthday, five years away. The date wasn't arbitrary. Statistics said I had a 67 percent chance of making it to 40 without a recurrence. My goal was simple: to build a life filled with all the things that cancer threatened or stole. Some of the things were little: Perfect my chocolate chip cookies, visit Graceland on my birthday. Some were simple but important: Get a good job with great benefits, have my own place again. Some were major: Climb Mt. Kilimanjaro, run the New York City Marathon.

My lemon saved my life because it showed me that this window, this parenthesis between birth and death, is all we have, and it matters what we do with it. The community of survivors who reminded me I wasn't alone in my struggle showed me that I could be, do, and imagine so much more than I thought I was capable of. For their love and support, I always will be grateful.

Over the next four years, I checked off each of those bucket-list items, one by one—yes, even Kilimanjaro. I reevaluated the list with every cancerversary and birthday, redefining my perfect life as I was living it. On my 40th birthday cake, the icing read: "Carpe Diem, Bitches." Five years after my last chemo treatment, I am living a life worth beating cancer for, and I could not be more thankful for the work it took to build it.

—April C., Colorado

From the Physical Pain of Multiple Sclerosis to Asymptomatic Health

Four years ago, with multiple sclerosis, my health was failing fast. I was in unbearable pain every single day. My mobility and strength were declining rapidly, and I felt utterly hopeless. I came across Dr. Terry Wahls's TED talk video. She, too, had advancing MS. Through extensive research, she developed a plan to reverse her symptoms and get her life back. Seeing her life transformation, I committed to following her plan in an attempt to garner similar results.

I eliminated all grains, refined sugars, legumes, dairy, and processed foods from my diet. I literally had dreams about pizza!

But I was determined. I read every single book on the subject and came to understand why certain foods had caused such an inflammatory response in my body, making it susceptible to an autoimmune disease.

Within two weeks, I started to feel like a different person. Within a month, I noticed that the oppressive daily pain began to ease. Within six months, I was in the gym doing light exercises—and it felt good! Within a year, I was participating in 5Ks! Within two years, I was nearly asymptomatic.

Twenty years ago, when I was diagnosed with MS, I was terrified. The struggles were many and oftentimes unbearable. Today, I honestly can say I am thankful for those struggles. Adversity made me strong. Multiple sclerosis was my lemon. Making huge changes to reverse my symptoms, finding my calling as a certified health and wellness coach, and dedicating my life to educating and bringing hope to others is my lemonade!

—Michele K., Texas

From Sterilizing Cancer Treatment to Motherhood and Helping Other Survivors Achieve Their Dreams of Parenthood

Receiving a breast cancer diagnosis at age 31 was definitely a lemon. But learning that chemotherapy would likely leave me infertile was the biggest, nastiest, rotting lemon I ever could imagine! The very idea that it might not be possible to become a mother, even though I was assured I would be cured of my stage 1 cancer, was far more devastating than the cancer diagnosis alone.

I spoke with a fertility specialist, who recommended preserving fertilized eggs (embryos) as my best chance for motherhood at the time. Then another lemon: preserving my fertility would cost $20,000! I didn't qualify for financial aid and, like 96 percent of the population, didn't have an extra $20,000 lying around. I handed my AMEX to the business manager and walked out with "fertility miles." Three days after my visit to the fertility clinic, I started a charity to ensure that other women didn't have the financial barrier to fertility preservation that I did.

As I was building our charity through chemo, I faced the darkest depression of my life, thanks to the treatment, three years of medical menopause, and serious financial issues. I was physically, mentally, and emotionally disabled. Getting better started with a few steps to the end of the block. Then around the block. Then down to the end of the street. Until finally I could walk a whole mile. With each step I took, I said the mantra, "Every day, in every way, we are getting better and better."

The charity grew. We formed community partnerships, raised money, and helped women realize their dreams of motherhood. But my own dream of motherhood hadn't yet come true. After four miscarriages, I finally heard my son's heartbeat on my five-year cancerversary. My charity, Fertile Action, is helping others make lemonade from their cancer diagnosis. My son turned my whole life into the sweetest, most delicious lemonade I ever could imagine.

For more about Fertile Action, visit fertileaction.org.

—Alice C., California

From Surviving Cancer Twice to Writing Tips and Tales for a Clean Lifestyle

I was diagnosed at age 31. It came out of left field. There was no family history and no side effects or signs, other than a lump. A mammogram revealed invasive ductal carcinoma. Breast cancer. It was horrifying to think of the what-ifs, but my husband and I were good cancer students. We shaved our heads, had chemo parties, and focused on the positives. We felt confident that cancer was a scary but closed chapter in our story.

I was proud that I gracefully smiled at surgery, chemo, and hair loss back then. I was even prouder when I jumped back into the corporate rat race. Unfortunately, my workaholic tendencies took me further away from taking care of myself. I bragged about waking up at 3 a.m. to send emails. I drank a week's worth of caffeine before 10 a.m. Too busy for lunch or a workout, I often ate low-fat potato chips from the vending machine, thinking I was eating "healthy."

It wasn't until I was diagnosed *again*, this time with stage 4 breast cancer, that I realized I needed to embrace my cancer life, not just look to get past it. I've always been passionate about health and fitness, so when I got the diagnosis of the second cancer, I used my resource-driven, organizational business skills, and got to work on figuring out my integrative health—aka cancer life plan—taking small steps to move toward wellness.

While I never wanted to be "that girl with cancer," my experiences and the lessons learned from them landed me with this powerful opportunity to help others realize that we can thrive even with a bad diagnosis. My message is about taking small steps to better your own health. I used to be that girl who was too busy to do anything. Now I write, post, and speak to that busy girl, the one who needs to take it one step at a time so that she can realistically implement change.

For more about my journey, visit prettywellness.com.

—Caryn S., Connecticut

GRATI'TUDE

All the stories on Gotta Make Lemonade take a seriously sour situation and turn it into something better through the power of positive mindset. This ongoing process of turning your thoughts from lemons to lemonade is what I call your grati'tude.

Here's an exercise to tone up your 'tude. Next time you sit down to dinner—with family, a friend, or support group—share one major blessing and one subtle beauty for the day.

Major Blessing

This is what you're most grateful for today. It's a biggie: your family, quality time at lunch with a girlfriend, the yoga instructor who totally turned your day around.

Example: "My family is such a major blessing. My kids gave me a huge, unsolicited hug as I came home from work today. Just what I needed after a stressful day."

Subtle Beauty

These babies are harder to spot, but when you look for them your day will get so much brighter. A subtle beauty puts a smile on your face, like a cute baby laughing, a goofy puppy, an awe-inspiring sunset, or a nice chat with the guy who bagged your groceries.

Example: "At spin class today, I got my favorite bike, the one right by the fan with a great view."

My family and I do this most nights at dinner. It may feel a little cheesy at first, but recognizing these big and little moments of positivity daily will change your day for the better and train your brain to see them as they happen.

GRATI'TUDE TRACKER

Use the chart at the right to track your 'tude for a week and then tell me on Twitter @samanthaharris how you feel.

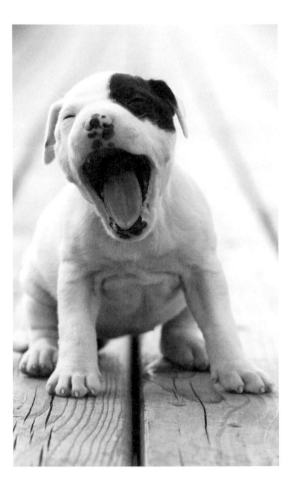

Day	Major Blessing	Subtle Beauty
Monday		
Tuesday		
Wednesday		
Thursday		
Friday		
Saturday		
Sunday		

YOUR HEALTHIEST ROAD MAP

Let's remember where we've been. Use this section as a handy-dandy guide to keep checking on yourself after you've finished the book. It's meant to stay with you, my healthy friend. Think about what you've read and try what you like and what sounds achievable. Then try a little more. After you've given yourself time to become the newer, healthier version of yourself, come back here to see what else you can add to your arsenal. That's exactly how I did it—slowly, just one or two small changes at a time. It won't happen overnight, but it sure *can* happen. We're in this together, and you can do it!

Remember that the path to your healthiest healthy is a journey. Take it one

1 ▸ Know Your Nutrition

Slash the sugar. Fill up with fiber. Avoid eating animals. Unleash your inner veggie. Load up on plant-based protein. Do your diligence on dairy. Make friends with healthy fats. Open your eyes to organic.

2 ▸ Wise Up Your Workout

Flex your motivation muscles. Find out what gets you moving and grooving. Change it up and keep it balanced for your muscles, heart, and mind. Focus on what your body can do, rather than how it looks.

3 ▸ Tame Your Toxins

Read those ingredients labels. Purge toxic products from your pantry, cabinets, drawers, and beauty bag.

4 ▸ Master Your Medical Mojo

Get up close and personal with yourself. Boost your Body IQ. Assemble an all-star doc squad and become your own best health advocate.

step at a time. Small steps add up to big changes, baby!

Scientists constantly are discovering and studying new things, so our exploration continues. Every day brings a new superfood to try or chemical ingredient to avoid. I'm staying on top of it, so don't worry: I'm not leaving you alone here! I'll continue distilling the latest research and sharing expert perspectives, encouragement, and inspiration for life's bitter moments. Join me on Twitter at @SamanthaHarris, on Instagram and Facebook at @SamanthaHarrisTV, and at YourHealthiestHealthy.com to stay current on the latest science that we can use together to keep the journey sweet.

5 **Handle Your Health**
Give yourself time to process health challenges. Communicate honestly and directly with your loved ones and your doc squad. Don't be afraid to ask for what you need.

6 **Get Real with Relationships**
Fire up your sweetest sex life. Make your healthiest healthy a fun family affair. Build your best support squad by doubling down on the Positive Pollys and nixing the Negative Nellys. Tap into the communities around you.

7 **Practice Positivity**
Pump your positive mindset by ditching negative thought patterns. Use your body to boost those positive vibes. Make time for meditation and mental breaks.

8 **Rev Your Resiliency**
Set process goals. Write them down. Practice your grati'tude. Own the voyage to your healthiest healthy.

THREE FINAL STEPS

We started with some small steps, so let's take a few more together in your victory lap!

STEP 1 **Celebrate your success.**

Put down this book, throw your hands in the air, and bask in your good-health glow, Wonder Woman–style! You've armed yourself with all the tools you need for a total health overhaul. Can I get a *woo-freakin'-hoo*? In all seriousness, applaud your commitment to your health and take pride in it, my healthy friend. Go on, do another booty shake. You've earned it!

STEP 2 **Post your goals.**

Take the goal sheet you created on pages 187–189 and put it somewhere that you'll see it. Reaching your healthiest healthy is about mastering your mindset and using all the tools in this book to reach your happiest, healthiest self every damn day. It's not about checking items off a list, moving on, and never looking back. These are lifestyle changes; you want them to last your whole, sweet life! Remember why you started and your intrinsic motivators. Take that positive energy and use it to move from one challenge to the next. Once you've mastered one goal, revisit this book to tackle the next one.

STEP 3 **Say it with me.**

I can do this.

I can't hear you. What was that?

I can do this!

There you go—now louder.

I CAN DO THIS!

That's right, my friend, you can. You are armed and ready to achieve your healthiest, happiest, most energized self. Take these tools and run with them. I'll see you back here again for your next step and then the next!

Ciao for now,

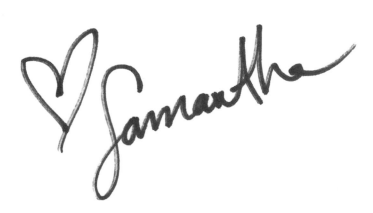

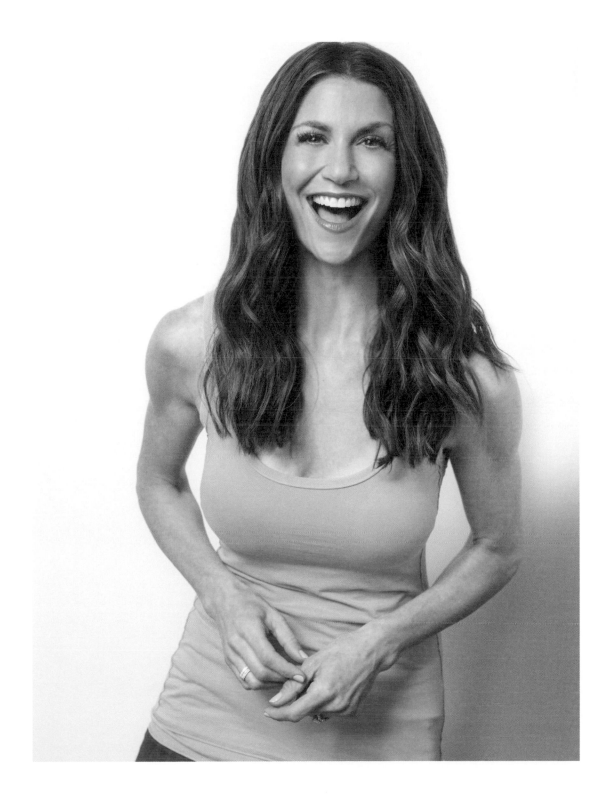

RESOURCES

CHAPTER 1. KNOW YOUR NUTRITION

Books

The Anti-Inflammation Zone by Barry Sears

The China Study, revised and expanded edition, by T. Colin Campbell and Thomas M. Campbell II

Crazy Sexy Diet by Kris Carr

Eat to Live by Joel Fuhrman

Food by Mark Hyman

Forks Over Knives by Gene Stone

How Not to Die by Michael Gregor and Gene Stone

The PlantPlus Diet Solution by Joan Borysenko

Apps & Websites

Fooducate.com A handy food tracker that translates nutrition label information and flags flimsy food choices.

Forksoverknives.com Dedicated to whole foods, plant-based nutrition, and education.

Habit.com Personalized nutrition tests to help you get to know your gut.

Ohmyveggies.com Yummy plant-based recipes to help you up your veggie intake.

PowerPerks, joinpowerperks.com Rachel Beller's online program has everything you need to know about nutrition and breast health, including all her tips and tricks to turn simple nutritional practices into lifelong habits.

Veganosity.com Vegan recipes with delicious variety.

Yummly.com Recipes, from a variety of sites, based on your preferences; specifies what to include or exclude.

CHAPTER 2. WISE UP YOUR WORKOUT

Books

Life As Sport by Jonathan Fader

The Telomere Effect by Elizabeth Blackburn and Elissa Epel

Apps & Websites

Livestrong.com Recipes, fitness tips, and inspiration for healthy living

CHAPTER 3. TAME YOUR TOXINS

Books

The Smart Human™ by Aly Cohen

Toxic Beauty by Samuel S. Epstein

Toxin Toxout by Bruce Lourie and Rick Smith

Apps & Websites

Credobeauty.com A great place to shop for beauty brands that are safe, clean choices.

Environmental Working Group, ewg.org, and specifically their **Healthy Living app,** which offers a handy way to scan barcodes to see what's in your food, cleaning, and beauty products, along with the corresponding ratings based on toxicity.

Lesstoxicguide.ca A Canadian environmental health guide that will help you spot toxic products and identify better-for-you alternatives.

Safecosmetics.org The Campaign for Safe Cosmetics (a project of Breast Cancer Prevention Partners) is your guide to cleaning out your personal care products.

Thedetoxmarket.com Similar to Credo Beauty; start shopping to update your beauty bag!

Think Dirty app Similar to EWG's Healthy Living app; rates beauty products based on toxicity.

CHAPTER 4. MASTER YOUR MEDICAL MOJO

Tools & Tests

Breast Cancer Risk Assessment Tool, cancer.gov/bcrisktool A tool from the National Cancer Institute that can help you determine your potential breast cancer risk.

Color Genomics, color.com This genetic testing company can screen specifically for cancer-related biomarkers.

Skinvision.com An app that helps you screen for skin cancer using your smartphone's camera.

Apps & Websites

American Cancer Society, cancer.org This website is your official headquarters for all things cancer-related, including info on risks and treatments.

Cancerschmancer.org Fran Drescher's initiative focuses on cancer prevention and early detection to save lives.

Lymphnet.org Learn more about your lymphatic system and find certified lymph specialists near you.

RateMDs.com Search more than 2 million doctor reviews and ratings to build an ace care team.

CHAPTER 5. HANDLE YOUR HEALTH

Books For Adults

How to Help Children through a Parent's Serious Illness by Kathleen McCue and Ron Bonn

Just Tell Me What to Say by Betsy Brown Braun

Raising an Emotionally Healthy Child When a Parent Is Sick by Paula K. Rauch and Anna C. Muriel

When a Parent Has Cancer by Wendy S. Harpham

Books For Kids

Nowhere Hair by Sue Glader (for ages 3–8)

When Your Parent Has Cancer by the National Cancer Institute (for teens)

The Year My Mother Was Bald by Ann Speltz (for ages 9–12)

CHAPTER 6. GET REAL WITH RELATIONSHIPS

Books

The Blue Zones by Dan Buettner

Love Worth Making by Stephen Snyder

Sex Rx by Lauren Streicher

Apps & Websites

Imermanangels.org Offers personalized connections that enable one-on-one support among cancer fighters, survivors, and caregivers.

Lookgoodfeelbetter.org Supports cancer patients by helping manage the appearance-related side effects of treatments.

Meetup.com

CHAPTER 7. PRACTICE POSITIVITY

Books

Positivity by Barbara L. Fredrickson

Presence by Amy Cuddy

Apps & Websites

Calm.com Guided meditations and oh-so-soothing natural scenes to clear your head when you're stuck at your desk. Also an app.

Headspace.com Hundreds of themed meditation sessions to help you practice your positivity.

CHAPTER 8. REV YOUR RESILIENCY

Books

Grit by Angela Duckworth

The Resilience Factor by Karen Reivich and Andrew Shatt

You Are a Badass by Jen Sincero

Apps & Websites

Gratefulness.io A daily prompt to share what you're grateful for each day, helping you build that grati'tude.

Happify.com A science-backed site and app to help form happier habits.

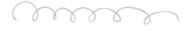

ACKNOWLEDGMENTS

Cancer sidelined me, but it didn't devour me. It ignited something so powerful that it compelled me to become healthier than ever and yearn to share the information, knowledge, and wisdom I gained along the way. Neither my life nor this book would be possible without a community of love and support. To all of you, I thank you from the depths of my heart. I am so incredibly grateful that you are in my life.

My Support Squad

My amazing hubby, Michael, for unwavering support, tenderness, and love; for guidance and positivity when moments of doubt strike; for being the most kick-ass teammate and partner for everything in life; for just "going with it" when I bring home yet another new plant-based recipe or "clean" shaving cream and toothpaste; and for being a rock-star daddy to our girls.

My girls, Jossie and Hilly, I couldn't be more proud of the young women you are blossoming into with thoughtfulness, compassion, awareness of optimal health, kindness, bursting personality, and not too many eye rolls when I ask you to eat your veggies. As I say every night, because of you, I'm the luckiest mommy ever.

My mom, Bonnie, you always said I would understand how much love you have for Aimée and me when I had kids of my own. There are no words to explain my gratefulness for all you've done and continue to do for us. Your love and generosity are infinite. Your guidance helped save my life and continues to be a beacon for so many aspects of my personal and professional life.

My daddy, "Richard the King," you are missed more than I ever could imagine. Forever you are in my heart. I wouldn't be who I am if it hadn't been for both you and Mommy. You are still and will always be the light of my being.

My sister, Aimée, for being my constant confidante and at my side in the hospital and in life; for being a role model as I watched you and tried to emulate everything you did when we were growing up; and for always being encouraging, compassionate, loving and there for me.

My Minneapolis family: my stepdad, Ricky, for being a great papa to our girls, for always being "on call" for us and for loving us as your own; Grandma Jackie for modeling healthful eating, exercise, and beauty from within; my stepsister, Katie; Max, Maddie, Michael, Auntie Patti and Uncle Michael, Auntie Andee and Uncle Bill, my cousins Sam, Cortney, Anthony, Jesse, and all my extended family, along with those who are part of my heart forever, including my best friends from high school, you know who you are—thank you for being there for me and always showing up.

My California-and-beyond family: Jeff, your generosity, love, and kindness know no bounds; Barbara and Bob, your love, support, and warmth are immeasurable; Chris "Stoph," Auntie Jan, cousin Suzanne, Sheila, my California friends, along with my college friends who helped me get through to the "other side" with texts, emails, phone calls, and laughter.

My Book Squad

Macaela Mackenzie, my fellow Northwestern University Medill School of Journalism alum, without whom *Your Healthiest Healthy* wouldn't be the beautiful book it is! For your dedication and your panache on the page. I couldn't have brought this book into the world without you, from your sharp eye for a story arc to your ability to bring readability to the latest research.

Stacey Glick, my literary agent, for believing in me and then in this book before its conception . . . and for not giving up!

James Jayo, my incredibly talented editor, and the team at Sterling Publishing, for taking a chance on a first-time author, guiding me, and championing *Your Healthiest Healthy* from proposal to finished product. It wouldn't sing without your conducting.

Rachel Beller, for your personal nutrition guidance, willingness to entertain even my silliest food questions, and just being so freakin' awesome and knowledgeable.

Meghan Coyle, my wonderful intern from the University of Southern California journalism school, for using your journalistic skills to research, locate, and hunt down contacts and for being so giving of your time.

My Medical Squad

Dr. Armando Giuliano, my mastectomy surgical oncologist, for your incredible skill at getting every last bit of the C-monster out of my body and for being a kick-ass part of making me cancer-free.

Dr. Dennis Slamon, my medical oncologist, for being the first onco to tell me I was going to live a long life, which calmed my fears. Your expertise as I continue on this journey, serving as the quarterback for my health care team, is beyond appreciated. Thank you as well for writing such a powerful and beautiful foreword to this book.

Dr. Cathie Chung, my medical oncologist, for being committed to giving me ongoing care as I continue with my healthiest life, truly empathizing with me as a patient, and really knowing your stuff.

Dr. Tiffany Grunwald, my reconstructive surgeon, for being with me every step of the way with warmth, support, top-notch skills, and incredible reassuring kindness even when things were crumbling around me. Oh yeah, and for giving me a really rockin' rack! (My hubby thanks you, too!)

Dr. Maureen Chung, my first surgical oncologist, who found my cancer, for listening to your gut when tissue-sample tests didn't detect invasive cancer—yet there it was in the final pathology. This saved my life.

Dr. Maggie DiNome, my current surgical oncologist, for being a champion in my ongoing care, always being literally a text away, and getting back to me at odd hours because of your incredible dedication to your patients!

Truly, thank you all. I love you.

IMAGE CREDITS

NOTES

CHAPTER 1: KNOW YOUR NUTRITION

1. https://www.ncbi.nlm.nih.gov/pmc/articles/PMC4940663/ http://jamanetwork.com/journals/jamainternalmedicine/fullarticle/2173094

2. https://www.cdc.gov/heartdisease/facts.htm

3. http://www.independent.co.uk/life-style/health-and-families/features/the-science-of-saturated-fat-a-big-fat-surprise-about-nutrition-9692121.html

4. http://www.independent.co.uk/life-style/health-and-families/features/the-science-of-saturated-fat-a-big-fat-surprise-about-nutrition-9692121.html

5. https://www.nytimes.com/2016/09/13/well/eat/how-the-sugar-industry-shifted-blame-to-fat.html?_r=0

6. https://www.sciencedaily.com/releases/2013/11/131114102528.htm

   http://onlinelibrary.wiley.com/doi/10.1002/oby.20460/abstract

   https://www.sciencedaily.com/releases/2013/08/130805131011.htm

   https://www.ncbi.nlm.nih.gov/pmc/articles/PMC3737458/

7. http://onlinelibrary.wiley.com/doi/10.1111/j.1574-0862.2012.00586.x/abstract

8. https://www.cdc.gov/obesity/adult/causes.html

9. https://health.gov/dietaryguidelines/2015/guidelines/appendix-2/

10. https://healthyforgood.heart.org/Eat-smart/Articles/Saturated-Fats

11. https://health.gov/dietaryguidelines/2015/guidelines/?linkId=20169028

12. http://ajcn.nutrition.org/content/97/4/677

13. http://www.health.harvard.edu/diseases-and-conditions/glycemic-index-and-glycemic-load-for-100-foods

14. http://jamanetwork.com/journals/jamainternalmedicine/fullarticle/1819573

    http://journals.plos.org/plosone/article?id=10.1371/journal.pone.0057873

15. https://www.ars.usda.gov/plains-area/gfnd/gfhnrc/docs/news-2013/dark-green-leafy-vegctables/

16. https://www.ncbi.nlm.nih.gov/pmc/articles/PMC3539819/

    http://ajph.aphapublications.org/doi/full/10.2105/AJPH.2016.303260

http://journals.plos.org/plosmedicine/article?id=10.1371/journal.pmed.1001878

http://www.bmj.com/content/349/bmj.g4490

17. http://www.onemedical.com/blog/live-well/retrain-palate/

18. http://www.mayoclinic.org/healthy-lifestyle/nutrition-and-healthy-eating/in-depth/fiber/art-20043983

19. https://health.gov/dietaryguidelines/2015/guidelines/appendix-7/

20. https://www.drfuhrman.com/learn/library/articles/13/fight-breast-cancer-with-flax-and-chia-seeds

21. https://www.hsph.harvard.edu/nutritionsource/what-should-you-eat/protein/

22. https://www.iarc.fr/en/media-centre/pr/2015/pdfs/pr240_E.pdf

23. http://nutritionstudies.org/the-china-study/

24. Eat to Live, Dr. Joel Fuhrman https://www.amazon.com/Eat-Live-Amazing-Nutrient-Rich-Sustained/dp/031612091X

25. http://jamanetwork.com/journals/jamainternalmedicine/article-abstract/2540540

26. http://www.bmj.com/content/349/bmj.g6015

27. http://nutritionstudies.org/provocations-dairy-protein-causes-cancer/

https://www.ncbi.nlm.nih.gov/pmc/articles/PMC4166373/

28. http://www.health.harvard.edu/staying-healthy/the-truth-about-fats-bad-and-good

29. https://www.choosemyplate.gov/2015-2020-dietary-guidelines-answers-your-questions

http://www.health.harvard.edu/staying-healthy/the-truth-about-fats-bad-and-good

30. http://www.nejm.org/doi/full/10.1056/NEJMra054035

31. https://www.ewg.org/foodnews/dirty_dozen_list.php

32. https://www.ewg.org/foodnews/clean_fifteen_list.php

CHAPTER 2: WISE UP YOUR WORKOUT

1. http://bmjopen.bmj.com/content/6/1/e007997

https://www.cancer.gov/about-cancer/causes-prevention/risk/obesity/physical-activity-fact-sheet#q6

https://internalmedicine.osu.edu/pulmonary/article.cfm?ID=3327

2. http://www.cell.com/current-biology/fulltext/S0960-9822(16)30465-1

3. http://journals.plos.org/plosone/article?id=10.1371/journal.pone.0131647

4. http://journals.plos.org/plosone/article?id=10.1371/journal.pone.0131647

5. http://www.cell.com/current-biology/fulltext/S0960-9822(16)30465-1

6. https://www.researchgate.net/publication/313291364_A_Self-Regulatory_Perspective_of_Work-to-Home_Undermining_SpilloverCrossover_Examining_the_Roles_of_Sleep_and_Exercise

7. https://www.ncbi.nlm.nih.gov/pubmed/25559067

8. http://www.sciencedirect.com/science/article/pii/S0005789416300119

9. http://www.sciencedirect.com/science/article/pii/S0005789416300119

10. https://www.sciencedaily.com/releases/2016/01/160118184354.htm

11. https://ijbnpa.biomedcentral.com/articles/10.1186/s12966-016-0437-z

12. https://www.eurekalert.org/pub_releases/2015-10/ppr-slh102315.php

13. https://www.ncbi.nlm.nih.gov/pubmed/25970659

14. https://www.ncbi.nlm.nih.gov/pubmed/23946713

15. https://www.ncbi.nlm.nih.gov/pubmed/18221285?dopt=Abstract

16. http://journals.plos.org/plosone/article?id=10.1371/journal.pone.0079342

17. https://www.ncbi.nlm.nih.gov/pmc/articles/PMC4122430/

18. https://www.ncbi.nlm.nih.gov/pubmed/12711737

19. https://www.ncbi.nlm.nih.gov/pubmed/21253795

https://www.ncbi.nlm.nih.gov/pubmed/19207713

https://www.ncbi.nlm.nih.gov/pubmed/21113764

20. https://internalmedicine.osu.edu/pulmonary/article.cfm?ID=3327

21. http://www.jmir.org/2015/8/e195/

22. http://www.onlinejacc.org/content/64/5/472

23. https://experiencelife.com/article/your-fitness-personality/

24. https://www.psychologytoday.com/files/attachments/34033/exercise-another.pdf

25. https://www.ncbi.nlm.nih.gov/pubmed/22395266

26. https://help.fitbit.com/articles/en_US/Help_article/1565#zones

27. http://www.tandfonline.com/doi/abs/10.1080/09658211.2014.889709

CHAPTER 3: TAME YOUR TOXINS

1. https://www.cancer.gov/about-cancer/causes-prevention/risk/myths/antiperspirants-fact-sheet#r3

   https://breast-cancer-research.biomedcentral.com/articles/10.1186/bcr2424

2. https://www.ncbi.nlm.nih.gov/pubmed/16045991

3. http://www.ewg.org/skindeep/2004/06/15/exposures-add-up-survey-results/

4. https://www.ncbi.nlm.nih.gov/pubmed/18484575

5. http://www.safecosmetics.org/get-the-facts/chemicals-of-concern/parabens/#sthash.YG1iTRfT.dpuf

6. https://ehp.niehs.nih.gov/14-09200/

   http://silentspring.org/research-update/lower-doses-common-product-ingredient-might-increase-breast-cancer-risk

   http://news.berkeley.edu/2015/10/27/lotion-ingredient-paraben-may-be-more-potent-carcinogen-than-thought/

7. https://www.ncbi.nlm.nih.gov/pubmed/16938376

8. https://www.ncbi.nlm.nih.gov/pubmed/11999442

9. https://draxe.com/phthalates/

   http://www.breastcancer.org/risk/factors/cosmetics

   https://www.ewg.org/skindeep/ingredient/702512/FRAGRANCE/#

10. http://articles.mercola.com/sites/articles/archive/2014/03/22/aluminum-toxicity-alzheimers.aspx

11. https://www.ewg.org/skindeep/ingredient/706623/TRICLOSAN/

12. https://www.ewg.org/skindeep/ingredient/702500/FORMALDEHYDE/

13. https://www.ewg.org/skindeep/ingredient/726331/1%2C4-DIOXANE/

14. http://www.safecosmetics.org/get-the-facts/chemicals-of-concern/14-dioxane/

    https://www.ncbi.nlm.nih.gov/pmc/articles/PMC4505343/

    http://davidsuzuki.org/issues/health/science/toxics/chemicals-in-your-cosmetics—-peg-compounds-and-their-contaminants/

15. https://www.ewg.org/skindeep/ingredient/706619/TRICETEARETH_4_PHOSPHATE/

16. http://www.safecosmetics.org/get-the-facts/chemicals-of-concern/petrolatum/

    https://www.ncbi.nlm.nih.gov/pmc/articles/PMC4677716/

17. https://www.ewg.org/skindeep/ingredient/704372/OXYBENZONE/

    http://www.ewg.org/sunscreen/report/the-trouble-with-sunscreen-chemicals/

18. http://www.safecosmetics.org/get-the-facts/chemicals-of-concern/ethanolamine-compounds/

19. http://www.safecosmetics.org/get-the-facts/chemicals-of-concern/coal-tar/

20. http://www.safecosmetics.org/get-the-facts/chemicals-of-concern/talc/

21. http://www.pesticideinfo.org/Detail_Chemical.jsp?Rec_Id=PC33019

22. https://www.ewg.org/skindeep/ingredient/704811/PHENOXYETHANOL/

23. http://www.safecosmetics.org/get-the-facts/chemicals-of-concern/retinol-and-retinol-compounds/

24. http://cur-lex.europa.eu/LexUriServ/LexUriServ.do?uri=OJ:L:2009:342:0059:0209:EN:PDF

    https://www.fda.gov/cosmetics/guidanceregulation/lawsregulations/ucm127406.htm

25. https://draxe.com/natural-skin-care/

26. http://www.huffingtonpost.com/thrive-market/olive-oil-and-hair-care_b_10972790.html

27. https://www.ellamila.com/blogs/in-the-news/115515716-5-toxic-chemicals-to-avoid-in-nail-polish

    https://www.ellamila.com/pages/7-free-nail-polish

28. https://www.atsdr.cdc.gov/phs/phs.asp?id=159&tid=29

    http://www.womensvoices.org/2015/05/18/nail-products-polishes-that-contain-chemicals-of-concern/#dbp

    http://nj.gov/health/eoh/rtkweb/documents/fs/0334.pdf

29. http://www.ewg.org/research/nailed#.WXayStPyuu4

    https://www.atsdr.cdc.gov/mmg/mmg.asp?id=291&tid=53

30. http://www.ewg.org/sunscreen/report/the-trouble-with-sunscreen-chemicals/#.WXauStPyuu4

31. http://www.ewg.org/sunscreen/report/the-trouble-with-sunscreen-chemicals/

    http://www.ewg.org/sunscreen/report/the-problem-with-vitamin-a/

    http://www.ewg.org/research/what-scientists-say-about-vitamin-sunscreen

32. http://www.womensvoices.org/wp-content/uploads/2013/11/Chem-Fatale-Report.pdf

33. http://time.com/4422774/tampons-toxic-cancer/

    http://www.agentorangerecord.com/information/what_is_dioxin/

34. http://www.who.int/mediacentre/factsheets/fs225/en/

35. http://www.cnn.com/2015/11/13/health/whats-in-your-pad-or-tampon/

36. http://www.womensvoices.org/wp-content/uploads/2013/11/Chem-Fatale-Report.pdf

37. http://www.huffingtonpost.com/2015/05/18/period-cost-lifetime_n_7258780.html

38. http://www.womensvoices.org/feminine-care-products/detox-the-box/always-pads-testing-results/

    http://www.cnn.com/2015/11/13/health/whats-in-your-pad-or-tampon/

39. https://ehjournal.biomedcentral.com/articles/10.1186/s12940-015-0043-6

40. https://www.govtrack.us/congress/bills/106/hr890/text

41. https://www.intimina.com/blog/whats-new-menstrual-cup-infographic/

42. http://www.figo.org/sites/default/files/uploads/News/Final%20PDF_8462.pdf

43. http://www.ewg.org/guides/cleaners/content/cleaners_and_health

44. https://www.cancer.org/cancer/cancer-causes/formaldehyde.html

45. https://www.epa.gov/sites/production/files/2014-03/documents/ffrro_factsheet_contaminant_14-dioxane_january2014_final.pdf

46. https://www.ncbi.nlm.nih.gov/pubmed/22034943

47. https://www.cdc.gov/niosh/ipcsneng/neng0061.html

48. https://medlineplus.gov/ency/article/002488.htm

49. http://www.nj.gov/health/eoh/rtkweb/documents/fs/0103.pdf

50. https://med.nyu.edu/pophealth/sites/default/files/pophealth/QACs%20Info%20for%20Physicians_18.pdf

51. https://www.cdc.gov/niosh/docs/81-123/pdfs/0256.pdf

52. https://toxtown.nlm.nih.gov/text_version/chemicals.php?id=22

53. https://toxtown.nlm.nih.gov/text_version/chemicals.php?id=24

54. http://www.ewg.org/guides/cleaners/content/top_products

55. http://articles.mercola.com/sites/articles/archive/2013/04/11/plastic-use.aspx

56. http://www.health.harvard.edu/staying-healthy/microwaving-food-in-plastic-dangerous-or-not

57. https://toxtown.nlm.nih.gov/text_version/chemicals.php?id=84

58. http://articles.mercola.com/sites/articles/archive/2013/04/11/plastic-use.aspx

59. https://www.atsdr.cdc.gov/phs/phs.asp?id=419&tid=74

 http://www.sciencedirect.com/science/article/pii/S1001074207600709

60. http://www.sciencedirect.com/science/article/pii/S1001074207600709

61. http://www.ewg.org/research/healthy-home-tips/tip-6-skip-non-stick-avoid-dangers-teflon

CHAPTER 4: MASTER YOUR MEDICAL MOJO

1. http://washingtonradiology.com/patient-education/breast-health-faq.asp

2. https://my.clevelandclinic.org/health/articles/breast-self-exam

3. https://www.aad.org/public/kids/skin/how-skin-grows

4. https://www.cancer.org/cancer/melanoma-skin-cancer/about/key-statistics.html

5. https://www.aad.org/public/spot-skin-cancer/learn-about-skin-cancer/detect

6. http://www.skincancer.org/skin-cancer-information/melanoma/melanoma-warning-signs-and-images/do-you-know-your-abcdes

7. http://articles.mercola.com/sites/articles/archive/2013/02/14/normal-stool.aspx

8. http://www.mayoclinic.org/stool-color/expert-answers/faq-20058080

9. http://www.sthk.nhs.uk/library/documents/stoolchart.pdf

10. http://articles.mercola.com/sites/articles/archive/2013/02/14/normal-stool.aspx

11. https://blogs.scientificamerican.com/lab-rat/what-makes-things-acid-the-ph-scale/

12. https://source.wustl.edu/2015/06/a-persons-diet-acidity-of-urine-may-affect-susceptibility-to-utis/

 https://draxe.com/balancing-act-why-ph-is-crucial-to-health/

13. https://www.ucsfhealth.org/tests/003583.html

14. https://draxe.com/balancing-act-why-ph-is-crucial-to-health/

15. http://www.clemson.edu/extension/food/food2market/documents/ph_of_common_foods.pdf

16. https://www.heart.org/HEARTORG/Conditions/HighBloodPressure/LearnHowHBPHarmsYourHealth/Health-Threats-From-High-Blood-Pressure_UCM_002051_Article.jsp

 http://www.heart.org/HEARTORG/Conditions/HighBloodPressure/LearnHowHBPHarmsYourHealth/How-High-Blood-Pressure-Can-Lead-to-Kidney-Damage-or-Failure_UCM_301825_Article.jsp#.WSCr0Wjyvb0

http://www.heart.org/HEARTORG/Conditions/HighBloodPressure/
LearnHowHBPHarmsYourHealth/How-High-Blood-Pressure-Can-Lead-to-Vision-Loss_
UCM_301826_Article.jsp#.WSCr92jyvb0

17. http://www.heart.org/HEARTORG/Conditions/HighBloodPressure/
LearnHowHBPHarmsYourHealth/How-High-Blood-Pressure-Can-Lead-to-Vision-Loss_
UCM_301826_Article.jsp#.WSCr92jyvb0

18. https://www.nhlbi.nih.gov/health/health-topics/topics/hbc

19. https://www.oxygenmag.com/fat-loss/the-fit-womans-guide-to-body-fat-9235

https://www.nhlbi.nih.gov/health/educational/lose_wt/risk.htm

20. https://books.google.com/books?id=CX8huSU0n8AC&pg=PA21&lpg=PA21&dq=dr+fuhrm
an+pinch+more+than+an+inch&source=bl&ots=ue54e5Se-P&sig=8E7eucofQaIfzCNRVEi6
DTDNmGc&hl=en&sa=X&ved=0ahUKEwj1mem99f7TAhXHTCYKHZpxCn4Q6AEIPzAF#v
=onepage&q=pinch&f=false

https://www.ncbi.nlm.nih.gov/pubmed/18362231?dopt=Citation

https://well.blogs.nytimes.com/2014/04/14/a-number-that-may-not-add-up/?_r=0

21. https://www.niddk.nih.gov/health-information/diabetes/overview/preventing-problems/
heart-disease-stroke

22. http://www.mayoclinic.org/tests-procedures/pap-smear/basics/why-its-done/prc-20013038

23. http://www.mayoclinic.org/tests-procedures/blood-pressure-test/basics/why-its-done/
prc-20020082

24. http://www.heart.org/HEARTORG/Conditions/Cholesterol/
HowToGetYourCholesterolTested/How-To-Get-Your-Cholesterol-Tested_UCM_305595_
Article.jsp#.WkrxdlT1Uxc

25. https://www.aace.com/files/final-file-hypo-guidelines.pdf

https://www.niddk.nih.gov/health-information/diagnostic-tests/thyroid

26. http://www.glaucoma.org/q-a/how-often-should-i-have-my-eyes-tested.php

27. http://www.mayoclinic.org/tests-procedures/mammogram/expert-answers/mammogram-
guidelines/faq-20057759

28. https://www.ghc.org/healthAndWellness/?item=/common/healthAndWellness/conditions/
diabetes/diagnosis.html

29. http://www.mayoclinic.org/tests-procedures/blood-pressure-test/basics/why-its-done/
prc-20020082

30. https://www.cancer.org/cancer/colon-rectal-cancer/detection-diagnosis-staging/acs-recommendations.html

31. https://www.nof.org/patients/diagnosis-information/bone-density-examtesting/

32. http://ww5.komen.org/BreastCancer/BreastCancerScreeningForWomenAtHigherRisk.html

33. https://medlineplus.gov/magazine/issues/winter07/articles/winter07pg17a.html

34. https://www.cancer.org/cancer/colon-rectal-cancer/causes-risks-prevention/risk-factors.html

35. https://www.aao.org/eye-health/diseases/glaucoma-risk

36. https://nihseniorhealth.gov/osteoporosis/riskfactors/01.html

37. https://www.cdc.gov/cancer/skin/basic_info/risk_factors.htm

38. https://www.womenshealthnetwork.com/community/askaquestion/thyroidhealth/thyroidtestingage.aspx

39. http://www.mayoclinic.org/diseases-conditions/diabetes/basics/risk-factors/con-20033091

40. http://health.usnews.com/health-news/health-wellness/articles/2015/11/10/many-patients-lie-to-their-doctors-survey-finds

41. http://healthaffairs.org/healthpolicybriefs/brief_pdfs/healthpolicybrief_86.pdf

CHAPTER 5: HANDLE YOUR HEALTH

1. http://www.pnas.org/content/112/28/8567.abstract

   http://news.stanford.edu/2015/06/30/hiking-mental-health-063015/

2. http://journals.lww.com/cancernursingonline/Abstract/2003/08000/An_Environmental_Intervention_to_Restore_Attention.5.aspx

3. Input from Rebecca Hendrix, LMFT.

4. Input from Ellen Jacobs, PhD.

5. Input from Ellen Jacobs, PhD.

CHAPTER 6: GET REAL WITH RELATIONSHIPS

1. https://www.ncbi.nlm.nih.gov/pubmed/15961213

   http://journals.plos.org/plosone/article?id=10.1371/journal.pone.0011597

   https://academic.oup.com/psychsocgerontology/article-lookup/doi/10.1093/geronb/gbx065

   http://www.nhs.uk/Livewell/Goodsex/Pages/ValentinesDay.aspx

2. http://www.nejm.org/doi/full/10.1056/NEJMoa067423#t=articleDiscussion

   http://www.nhs.uk/Livewell/Goodsex/Pages/ValentinesDay.aspx

3. https://www.ncbi.nlm.nih.gov/pmc/articles/PMC2854915/

4. T. Colin Campbell, PhD, and Thomas M. Campbell II, MD, *The China Study*, revised and expanded ed., pp. 76, 77, 154.

5. https://ijbnpa.biomedcentral.com/articles/10.1186/s12966-017-0509-8

   http://journals.plos.org/plosmedicine/article?id=10.1371/journal.pmed.1000316

6. http://interpersona.psychopen.eu/article/view/162/html

   http://www.elainehatfield.com/ch50.pdf

7. http://irep.ntu.ac.uk/id/eprint/27260/

CHAPTER 7: PRACTICE POSITIVITY

1. https://www.ncbi.nlm.nih.gov/pmc/articles/PMC3156028/

2. https://www.ncbi.nlm.nih.gov/pmc/articles/PMC3156028/

3. https://www.ncbi.nlm.nih.gov/pmc/articles/PMC1693418/

4. https://www.ncbi.nlm.nih.gov/pubmed/23967061

5. http://www.sciencedirect.com/science/article/pii/S0747563214005767

   http://munews.missouri.edu/news-releases/2015/0203-if-facebook-use-causes-envy-depression-could-follow/

6. https://www.ncbi.nlm.nih.gov/pmc/articles/PMC474733/

   http://www.apa.org/monitor/2011/12/exercise.aspx

7. https://www.ncbi.nlm.nih.gov/pmc/articles/PMC3193654/

   http://jandonline.org/article/S0002-8223(09)00628-2/fulltext

   https://www.sciencedaily.com/releases/2009/08/090803185712.htm

8. https://www.ncbi.nlm.nih.gov/pmc/articles/PMC3193654/

9. http://datacolada.org/wp-content/uploads/2015/05/Carney-Cuddy-Yap-2010.pdf

10. http://datacolada.org/wp-content/uploads/2015/05/5110-Ranehill-Dreber-Johannesson-Leiberg-Sul-Weber-PS-2015-Assessing-the-robustness-of-power-posing-no-effect-on-hormones-and-risk-rolerance-in-a-large-sample-of-men-and-women.pdf

11. http://journals.sagepub.com/doi/abs/10.1177/0956797614553946

12. https://www.ncbi.nlm.nih.gov/pmc/articles/PMC3156028/

13. http://www.sciencedirect.com/science/article/pii/016383439500025M

14. http://psychnet.apa.org/journals/str/12/2/164/

15. http://www.sciencedirect.com/science/article/pii/S0376871616001174

16. https://www.ncbi.nlm.nih.gov/pmc/articles/PMC3090218/

17. http://www.nature.com/tp/journal/v6/n8/full/tp2016164a.html

18. http://www.sciencedirect.com/science/article/pii/S0889159112004758

19. https://www.ncbi.nlm.nih.gov/pmc/articles/PMC4999800/

    https://www.ncbi.nlm.nih.gov/pmc/articles/PMC4410786/

    https://www.ncbi.nlm.nih.gov/pmc/articles/PMC3612673/

20. https://www.ncbi.nlm.nih.gov/pubmed/19568835

CHAPTER 8: REV YOUR RESILIENCY

1. https://www.ncbi.nlm.nih.gov/pmc/articles/PMC4346032/

2. https://www.ncbi.nlm.nih.gov/pmc/articles/PMC4346032/

3. http://journals.sagepub.com/doi/abs/10.1177/0146167299025002010

4. http://www.dominican.edu/academics/ahss/undergraduate-programs/psych/faculty/assets-gail-matthews/researchsummary2.pdf

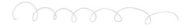

INDEX

Toxins, 71–99. *See also* Household products; Personal care products
    in cleaning products, 90–92
    healthy alternatives to, 80–90, 94–96
    Keep-Off-Your-Bod List, 76–77
    in personal care products, 71–78
    in plastics, 96–99
Trans fats, 21, 42
Type 2 diabetes, 120

U

University of California at Berkeley, studies at, 74
Urine, 112–113

V

Vegetables. *See also* Recipes
    increasing intake of, 23
    in smoothies, 24

W

Wahls, Terry, 191
Waist circumference, 117
Weight loss, 47
Women's Voices for the Earth, 87

Workout, 49–69
    exercising during pregnancy, 67
    for families, 164–166
    for fitness, 55–57
    heart rate zones for, 68
    log for, 69
    for lymphatic system, 114
    measuring effort and, 68–69
    motivation for, 49–51, 53–54, 57–58
    peak shape with, 51–53
    positivity for physical health and, 176–179
    preventing injuries and, 66–68
    for self-care during crises, 137
    strategies for, 59–66
World Health Organization, 30, 87

Y

Yale University, study by, 96
Yoga
    for introverts, 64
    meditation and, 179–183
    for positivity, 176–178
    Power Posing, 179
Yogurt, reducing in diet, 41
YourHealthiestHealthy.com, 179

ABOUT THE AUTHOR

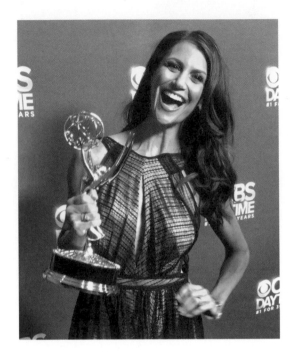

SAMANTHA HARRIS is an Emmy-winning television host and breast cancer survivor. She cohosted *Dancing with the Stars* for eight seasons, garnering two Emmy nominations, and served as correspondent and weekend anchor on *Entertainment Tonight*, where she earned two more Emmy nominations and a win. She has hosted dozens of other programs, including *E! News*, *Extra*, and *The Insider*, and has appeared as a guest host on *Access Hollywood Live*, *The View*, and *Who Wants to Be a Millionaire?* She cohosted the official live red carpet show for the 80th Academy Awards, and she made her Broadway debut in *Chicago* in 2009. A certified personal trainer, she has appeared on the covers of numerous health and fitness magazines, including *Muscle & Fitness HERS* (a record four times) and *Shape*, and she has been featured in the pages of *Health*, *People*, *SELF*, *Star*, *US Weekly*, and *USA Today* magazine. Named Survivor of the Year by Susan G. Komen Race for the Cure Los Angeles, she led the 2018 Parade of Promise at Dodgers Stadium and also serves as a spokesperson for the American Cancer Society. She founded the online community GottaMakeLemonade.com to inspire positivity in the face of adversity. She lives in Southern California with her husband and their two daughters. Visit her @SamanthaHarris on Twitter, @SamanthaHarrisTV on Facebook and Instagram, and at samantha-harris.com.

DENNIS SLAMON, MD, serves as director of clinical/translational research and as director of the Revlon/UCLA Women's Cancer Research Program at the Jonsson Comprehensive Cancer Center. He is a professor of medicine, chief of hematology/oncology, and executive vice chair for research for the Department of Medicine at the University of California at Los Angeles. He also serves as director of the Medical Advisory Board for the National Colorectal Cancer Research Alliance. Dr. Slamon and his colleagues conducted the laboratory and clinical research that identified HER2-positive breast cancer and led to the development of Herceptin. President Clinton appointed him to the three-member President's Cancer Panel in 2000. Dr. Slamon has won numerous awards honoring his scientific endeavors, including: the American Cancer Society Medal of Honor, the Bristol-Myers Squibb Oncology Millennium Award, the David A. Karnofsky Memorial Award from the American Society of Clinical Oncology, the European Institute of Oncology Breast Cancer Award, the Gairdner Foundation International Award, and the Warren Alpert Foundation Scientific Prize from Harvard Medical School. He lives in Southern California.